Agrotechniques of
Medicinal Plants

Agrotechniques of
Medicinal Plants

R.C. Upadhyaya

ANMOL PUBLICATIONS PVT. LTD.
NEW DELHI-110 002 (INDIA)

ANMOL PUBLICATIONS PVT. LTD.
H.O.: 4374/4B, Ansari Road, Darya Ganj,
New Delhi-110 002 (India)
Ph.: 23278000, 23261597

B.O.: No. 1015, Ist Main Road, BSK IIIrd Stage
IIIrd Phase, IIIrd Block
Bangalore - 560 085 (India)
Visit us at: www.anmolpublications.com

Agrotechniques of Medicinal Plants

First Published, 2008

ISBN 978-81-261-3421-2

PRINTED IN INDIA

Printed at Mehra Offset Press, Delhi.

Contents

Preface *vii*

1. **Introduction** **1**
Commonly Used Medicinal Plants • Conservation and Development of Medicinal Plants • Schemes of Different Agencies • Cultivation of Medicinal Plants • Research and Development of Medicinal Plants

2. **Herbalism** **49**
Coffee

3. **Medicinal Plants in Alternative Medicine** **65**

4. **Medicinal Plants in Ayurveda** **79**
Home Remedies - Siddha, Ayurveda & Unani

5. **Medicinal Plants and Phytomedicines** **93**
Products Involved in Plant Ecophysiology • The Benefits of Phytomedicines • A Perspective on Five Medicinal Plants • Conclusions and Outlook • DNA Microarrays in Herbal Drug Research • DNA Microarrays in Pharmacogenomics

6. **Guidelines for Medicinal Plants** **129**
Guidelines for Good Agricultural Practice • Medicinal Plants • MedicinalPlants of Meru • Medicinal Plants—Industrial Profiles • New Support for Medicinal Plants • Medicinal Plants and CITES • Market Segments • Current and Potential Production • Quantities by Products

• Description of Producers • Competition between the Suppliers • International Trade in Medicinal Plants

7. **Sustainable Use of Medicinal Plants** **215**
A Multi-sectoral Challenge • Developing the Medicinal Plants • Medicinal Plants—The Global View • Considering the Role for India • Industry Roles in Medicinal Plant Conservation • Exporting Company—Pukka Herbs • Medicinal Plants

Bibliography 255

Index 261

Preface

Horticulture has a special significance for the economic development. Most of the people, though hard working and face the calamities of nature and live in harsh conditions, yet produce lot of fruits, vegetables and other flowering and ornamental plants including the medicinal and aromatic plants. In order to increase the productivity of horticultural crops growers must take the advantage of the expertise of scientists. Keeping this idea in focus, the present work has been compiled which contains experiences of the experts and related people. The volumes cover advances in strategies, production, plant protection, value addition and other important areas of horticulture development.

The Encyclopaedia provides practical information on production technologies of tropical and subtropical fruits as well as plantation crops and horticultural nursery. Post-harvest management, marketing and export trends have been furnished for guidance. It also presents most realistic cost estimates and returns from cultivation of such crops. The volumes aim at viewing commercial prospects for horticulture. It has been carefully designed to meet the queries of intending investors, financial institutes, creditors, traders and growers engaged in dealing with horticultural crops. Further it will serve the purpose reference books to students, academicians and related people.

R.C. Upadhyaya

1

Introduction

There has been a resurgence in the consumption and demand for medicinal plants. These plants are finding use as pharmaceuticals, neutraceuticals, cosmetics and food supplements. Even as traditional source of medicines and they continue to play pivotal rule.

The World Health Organisation (WHO) estimated that 80% of the population of developing countries still relies on traditional medicines, mostly plant drugs, for their primary health care needs. Also, modern pharmacopoeia contains at least 25% drugs derived from plants. Many other are synthetic analogues built on prototype compounds isolated from plants. Demand for medicinal plant is increasing in both developing and developed countries due to growing recognition of natural products, being non-toxic, having no side-effects, easily available at affordable prices. Medicinal plant sector has traditionally occupied an important position in the socio-cultural, spiritual and medicinal arena of rural and tribal lives of Tamil Nadu.

Millions of rural households use medicinal plants in a self-help mode. Over 20,000 practitioners of the Indian System of Medicine in the oral and codified streams use medicinal plants in preventive, promotive and curative applications in Tamil Nadu. There are estimated to be about 1000 manufacturing units in Tamil Nadu.

In recent years, the growing demand for herbal product has led to a quantum jump in volume of plant materials traded within and across the countries. An estimate of the EXIM Bank puts the international market of medicinal plants related trade at US$ 60 billion per year growing at the rate of 7% only.

Though India has a rich biodiversity, the growing demand is putting a heavy strain on the existing resources. While the demand for medicinal plants is growing, some of them are increasingly being threatened in their natural habitat. For meeting the future needs cultivation of medicinal plant has to be encouraged.

According to an all India ethno biological survey carried out by the Ministry of Environment & Forests, Government of India, there are over 8000 species of plants being used by the people of India.

Culture & History of Siddha Medicine: The science of medicine is of fundamental importance to man's well being and his survival, and so it must have originated with man and developed as civilization advanced. It is therefore rather pointless to try to determine the exact point of time when any system of medicine was evolved and codified. A system of medicine is not a discovery but a gradual evolution during successive periods of history. It owes its progress to great men, who have not only enriched the science, but also society and civilization as a whole.

There are two ancient systems of medicine in India, the Siddha that flourished in the South and the Ayurveda prevalent in the North. Instead of giving the name of any one individual as the founder of either system, our ancients wisely attributed their origin to the Creator. According to tradition, it was Shiva who unfolded the knowledge of Siddha system of medicine to his consort, Parvati, who handed it down to Nandideva and he, to Siddhars.

Therefore it is called 'Saiva Sampradayam' (tradition of Shive), or 'Siddha Sampradayam'. In the case of Ayurveda it was Brahma, the Creator of the Universe, who taught the science to Prajapati, he to Ashwini Devatas and they, in their turn, to Atreya etc. So this tradition is called the Brahma or Arsha Sampradaya (the tradition of Rishis). The inference to be drawn from these traditions is that, there is no exact point of time to which the beginning of these systems could be traced. They are eternal, without a beginning or end; they began with man.

The Tamils have a distinct civilization, which is not disputed by historians. The recorded history of the Tamils is thousands of years old. Apart from the literature of the first, the middle and the last Sangam periods which bears ample testimony to the extent of Tamil civilization and its eminence, mention is made even in contemporary Sanskrit literature about Cholas, Pandiyas and Cheras and their kingdoms. A civilized society must naturally have had a system of medicine which catered to the health needs of its people. This was the Siddha system. The term 'Siddhi' means 'achievement' and the Siddhars were men who achieved certain results in medicine, as well as in yoga or tapas. The results in medicine were achieved by the Siddhars through their mental powers, they bequeathed to their 'Chilas' or pupils, who preserved and propagated the science.

Eighteen siddhas seem to have existed. They should have lived at different periods and bequeathed their experiences in medicine and yoga to posterity. The names of these eighteen Siddhas differ from one source to another. It is not necessary to dogmatise which of these enumerations is correct. Some of the Siddhas, for example, Kapila and Kakabujanda have written treatises both in Tamil and in Sanskrit. It is possible that the originals were written in Tamil and that they were translated into Sanskrit later.

The following is the list of eighteen Siddhas according to one recension: 1. Nandi 2. Agasthiyar 3. Thirumular 4. Punnakkeesar 5. Pulasthiyar 6. Poonaikannar 7. Idaikadar 8. Bogar 9. Pulikai Isar 10. Karuvurar 11. Konkanavar 12. Kalangi 13. Sattainathar 14. Azhuganni 15. Agappai 16. Pambatti 17. Theraiyar and 18. Kudhambai.

Names like Bogar, Idaikadar and Theraiyar are of recent origin and these Siddhars lived probably in the middle ages. There are also authors of Siddha treatises like Sattaimuni, Yugimuni, Macha Muni, Kakabusundar etc., whose works are available in parts at the present day and are being used.

Distribution of Medicinal plants in Tamil Nadu: Analysis of habits of medicinal plants indicates that they are distributed across various habitats. One third are trees and an equal portion shrub and the remaining one-third herbs, grasses and climbers. A very small proportion of the medicinal plants are lower plants like lichens, ferns algae, etc. Majority of the medicinal plant are higher flowering plants.

The State of Tamil Nadu is endowed with a very rich flora. Due to the various physiographic features and physiognomic factors, different types of vegetation exists in the state: 1. Coastal vegetation; 2. Island vegetation; 3. Vegetation of hills and mountains comprising of:

(1) Dry deciduous forests
(2) Moist deciduous forests
(3) Semi-evergreen forests
(4) Wet evergreen forests
(5) Sholas (Southern montane wet temperate forests)

The altitude varies from sea level to 2637 m including the well known mountain ranges—the Nilgiri, the Anamalais and the Cardamom hills which harbours different types of ecological niches, ecosystem and innumerable medicinal plants. A few ethnic tribes like the Irular, Kaanikkara, Karumpar, Palliyan, Paniyar, Sholagar, Thodar and others dwell in these ecosystems and still depend on naturally occurring or cultivated from the state (N.C. Nair & A.N Henry, Flora of Tamil Nadu, India,-Analysis—Vol. I, 1983, B.S.I., Coimbatore). Out of this, it is found that 1474 are medicinal plants. A total number are found to be used in Siddha system of medicine which is commonly practiced throughout the state.

Tampcol has two medicinal farms, one in Chennai city at Arumbakkam and at Valavandinadu, Kolli hills, Namakkal district. In Chennai farm six varieties of medicinal plants are cultivated in five acres to meet the fresh herb requirements for the production of herbal hair tonic, other medicated oils and also supplied to pharmacy at Arignar Anna Govt. Hospital for Indian medicine and Homoeopathy, Chennai.

Another 150 varieties of medicinal plants are maintained in the parts as reference material. The farm is also visited by the students of all systems of Indian Medicine. Leading practitioners of Indian Medicine also make use of this farm as their reference for medicinal plants. This farm is very popular and has contributed for herbal awareness in Chennai City. The farm participates in the exhibitions conducted by Educational Institutions, Trade fairs and seminars/conferences in the city. The public are also encouraged to buy the medicinal plants at low prices to enhance the importance and awareness of herbal medicines.

The Kolli Hills medicinal farm is situated in Valavandinadu at the altitude of 3600 ft. The land is undulating with rocky slopes. Out of 105 acres year-marked, the corporation has developed 55 acres and cultivating a dozen species of medicinal plants on large scale and another 50 varieties which includes trees, climbers, perennials are cultivated on bunds, hedges, fence line etc. as per suitability of the species. Further, the farm has a large nursery in which seedlings/saplings/cuttings/graftings are raised for own cultivation and to supply to the government institutions concerned and also to progressive farmers in the state and out side.

Raw Drugs Trading: The corporation is handling 400 varieties of raw drugs of plant, metal/mineral, animal and marine origin for the production of its own products and to supply to four government pharmacies of ISM in the state and also for the outside sales. The corporation is well worsed in the All India raw drug trade and can source raw drugs for domestic and overseas markets.

Tampcol Products: The corporation has been manufacturing 50 medicines of Siddha, Ayurveda and Unani systems and supplying to all the ISM wings, in PHC's/Dispensaries/Hospitals and Taluk/District hospitals in the state of Tamil Nadu apart from supplying to TNEB dispensaries and CGHS dispensaries in Chennai city. The products are also sold in the open market through dealers and Tampcol's outlets in Chennai and Palayamkottai .

Medicinal Plants

I. *Definition:* Plants used for healing purposes.

II. *Uses of Medicinal Plants:* Medicinal plants can:

1. be used intact to make a tea, or poultice, etc. This is

the pattern in herbal and traditional medicine. An advantage of using the intact plant is that several different components in the plant may act together (synergistically) to produce the desired effect;

2. serve as the source of a drug that is extracted and purified from the plant. This is the typical situation in Western medicine. Advantages of extracting the drugs - dose is more easily controlled; sale of the product is also controlled (via patents);
3. serve as the starting material for the synthesis of other drugs (*i.e.*, Mexican yam, periwinkle), or
4. serve as the model of the synthesis of novel new drugs.

III. Importance of herbal medicines.

Medicinal plants are a very important component of the US. Pharmacopoeia. For example, between 1959-1973, 25% of all prescription drugs in US contained one or more substances from plants as the active ingredient. In 1973, approximately 1.03 billion dollars was spent on these drugs. Interestingly, in 1974 the American pharmaceutical industry spent one billion dollars on research, yet only 200,000 for research on drug plants.

IV. Pharmacognosy.

Study of medicines obtained from plants:

V. Brief History of Medicinal Plants.

- Western medicine originates with the Greeks.
    - o Hippocrates (460-377 BC)—Founder of medicine
    - o Aristotle—was a great natural historian
    - o Theophrastus (372-287 BC)—Founder of botany, described many plants
    - o Pliny (43-70 AD)—major compendium of natural history
    - o Dioscorides (40-90 AD)—De Materia Medica-encyclopedia of medicinal plants that was major gospel of plant medicine form hundreds of years. Information was accepted probably cuz of:

(a) series of wars; (b) Black Death; (c) hi infant mortality (60%). During this time, monasteries were pockets of scholarship. They produced herbals, but mostly copied faithfully info from past. Fortunately the Arabs (*i.e.*, Avicenna) filled the intellectual void. The trend wasn't reversed until the printing press made information available outside of monasteries and the advent of the Renaissance.

- Gerard's Herbal
- Herbal medicine eventually gave way to more scientific studies. From the Greek notion that pure reason could answer any question, empirical studies developed.
- Herbal medicines in other cultures. Herbs are very important components of medicine in other cultures (*i.e.*, Chinese medicine; Indian Ayurvedic medicine; native North American Indians).

VI. Drug Discovery or, how did our ancestors learn which plants were useful for medicinal purposes?

1. Trial and error. The original experiments with medicinal plants. Our ancestors tried different plants until one seemed to work. Over time this served to empirically test the validity of many herbal remedies.
2. Superstitions/Religious Beliefs. It is likely that religious beliefs also played an early role in the discovery of medicinal plants. Disease was thought to be caused by spirits. Since disease was bad, it followed that you could cure the disease if you eat something that tastes bad (bitter). Using this logic may have sometimes paid off because as it turns out, many bitter-tasting plants contain alkaloids or other biologically-active chemicals.
3. Doctrine of Signatures (Paracelsus; 1493-1524)-suggested that God provided clues about the medicinal value of a plant in the plant's general form. Thus, walnuts were thought to be good "brain food" and

bloodroot good for circulatory problems. Scientists disregard this idea, though many traditional healers still accept it.

VII. Drug Discovery in the 21st Century.

In general, there is a modern prejudice against herbal drugs/medicines. This is partly the result of our love of new technology and our cultural prejudices (*i.e.*, "witch doctor"). Fortunately, this is changing for a variety of reasons: (a) concerns over loss of global biodiversity; (b) increased cultural sensitivity; (c) new tools in the laboratory to help in the screening process; and (d) better incentives (*i.e.*, economic, social, political, other). The general steps for identifying medicinal plants is:

A. Identify Potential Medicinal Plants

1. Random Approach - plants are selected more-or-less at random. Taxol, used to treat breast cancer, was discovered this way.
2. Targeted Search - plants with "promising" activity are screened for activity. Plants are selected on the basis of: (a) Phylogeny - plants related to those with known medicinal activity are studied; and (b) cultural pre-screen - plants known to be used medicinally by indigenous cultures are studied. This latter method can be accomplished by checking the literature for reports of plants used by people; studying the herbarium for information about medicinal plants; or visiting and conducting studies of other cultures. This is one of the jobs of an "ethnobotanist." Richard Evans Schultes and Mark Plotkin are good examples of ethnobotanists who have extensively studied the medicinal (and other plants) of South American natives. Good ones, like Plotkin and Schultes, must know the language of the people, must develop a working relationship, understand the culture, obtain direct exposure to the culture (participant observer, not just an objective observer), recreated experiences.

B. Botanical Investigations.

As much as possible is learned about the plant. It is collected and voucher specimens are preserved (in a herbarium). Appropriate permissions must first be obtained and the ethnobotanist must negotiate an equitable return for the country/people involved.

C. Screening for Biologically Activity.

The plant is extracted and the extract is tested for biological activity with a bioassay. A bioassay is a test that examines the effect of a test chemical on a living system. There are many bioassays. We will perform two bioassays in lab using brine shrimp and the bacterium, Escherischia coli. The use of animals is now avoided.

D. Chemically Analyze the Extract.

If the extract shows biological activity in the screening tests, the extract is fractionated (separated into individuals components) and then each fraction is tested for activity to isolate and identify the active ingredient(s).

E. Synthesis.

Once the biodynamic chemical has been isolated and identified, it will be synthesize so that enough will be available for further testing and use. In some cases, the chemical cannot be synthesized, so it must be extracted from a natural source.

F. Clinical Trials.

Phase I - Toxicity Studies; Phase II - Efficacy in Small Groups; Phase III - Large scale study, double blind.

VII. Survey of Select Medicinal Plants - we will study several medicinal plants. As we consider each plant, we will focus on five major concepts:

1. Folk Use & History - how was the plant used by native/indigenous people? Is it still used this way?
2. Scientific Discovery - how did knowledge of the medicine come to the attention of scientists (ethnobotanists)?
3. Botanical Explorations - what do we know about the plant? where does it grow? What parts are used? etc.

4. Physiological Action of the Plant - what is the action of the plant on humans?
5. Chemical Explorations - what are the active ingredients? what kind of molecules are they? how do they act?

VIII. Foxglove (Digitalis purpurea)

Folk Use/History: Used by an old woman from Shropshire to treat dropsy - which is caused by an accumulation of fluid (lungs, abdomen, extremities), which in turn, is due to a failure of heart to pump properly. One of the components of her mixture was foxglove.

Scientific Discovery: William Withering learned about this folk remedy plant about 1775. He was an English country doctor and good botanist.

Botanical Explorations: This plant is a biennial in the Snapdragon family (Scrophulariaceae). It had been listed in Gerard's herbal as a powerful medicinal plant.

Physiological Activity: Withering found it successful in treating dropsy. Published account of his studies. One problem was with dosage. Amount varied with season, etc.

Chemical Explorations: Foxglove provides about 30 different steroidal glycosides including digoxin & digitonin. These chemicals are powerful heart drugs. Stimulate heart muscle. Slows rate of heart beat and increases the strength of each beat. Not yet commercially synthesized - still extracted from foxglove leaves.

IX. Snakeroot (Rauwolfia serpentina)

Folk Use/History: Used for centuries in India to treat snakebite because of the snakelike appearance of root. Also used to cure "madness", put child to sleep (cure insomnia) and treat anxiety.

Scientific Discovery: Ignored for years; slowly accepted and studied.

Botanical Explorations: Named and identified in eighteenth century.

Physiology & Chemistry: In 1930's, Indian chemists isolated molecules, relatively inactive. Another student showed powder had hypnotic effect and lowered blood pressure. In 1949 two chemists at CIBA in Basel isolated reserpine and found it had strong activity. Alkaloid. Blocks neurotransmitter, acts on hypothalamus.

X. Aspirin.

Folk Use/History: The bark of the willow has long been used as a pain reliever by Greeks as well as native Americans-independent discoveries.

Scientific Discovery: Important plant in Gerard's herbal.

Botanical Explorations: Found in willow (Salix), meadowsweet (Spiraea or Filipendula ulmaria) and wintergreen.

Physiological Explorations : Early studies by Rev Edmund Stone found the bark was good for fever and chills. Effects - anti-inflammatory, antipyretic (reduces fever); analgesic (reduces pain). Major effect by suppressing the release of prostaglandins that are released by injured cells (also stimulated by other hormones). Also shown to reduce risk of heart attack/stroke due to its ability to suppress aggregation of blood platelets that could form blood clots.

Chemistry: French & German chemists worked on isolating active ingredients. In 1828 isolated salicin (a glycoside of salicylic acid). Lead to the lab synthesis of salicylic acid. In 1898 Felix Hoffmann at Bayer Co. learned about a derivative- acetylsalicylic acid - more effective, fewer side effects (stomach irritation). Named it aspirin (a = acetylsalicylic acid; spirin = Spirea).

XI. Fever Bark Tree (Cinchona sp.)

Folk Use/History/Scientific Discovery: Used to treat malaria. This disease has probably killed more people than all wars and plagues and Black Death. Even today, there is a very high rate of death. Caused by protozoan parasite (Plasmodium) transmitted by a mosquito. People didn't originally know the cause, thought it was caused by bad air (mal aria, Italian). Killed thousands during the Civil War, as far north as St. Louis, and even Minnesota. The fall of Rome and Greece were due in part to malaria. During WWII, one half of all troops suffered from malaria.

Used by Peruvian Indians to treat fevers. Gave plant the name quina.

Discovered during the conquest of the Incan Empire in the late 16th and early 17th century. Spanish legends indicate a soldier suffering from malaria drank from a pool of brown water at base of quinine tree. Another Spanish legend suggests that Indians noted sick animals drinking water from the brown tepid pools.

Word of Cinchona reached Europe in 1630's by Jesuits. Worked great. But, physicians were wary of using it because: (a) it was new; (b) sponsored by the Jesuits - feared it was a plot by Catholics to kill Protestants. For example, Oliver Cromwell died rather than being "Jesuited to death".

Robert Talbor, apothecary, used quinine in a secret remedy to cure malaria. Cured the Royal family (Charles II) also the ailing son of Louis XIV. He was knighted. He was rather clever because he belittled Peruvian bark, but kept his recipe a secret until his death. His recipe included rose leaves, lemon juice, cinchona bark.

Struggle for bark in the 1800's. S. America wanted to keep its monopoly. Prohibited export. Tried to smuggle seeds/cuttings. Quinine was critical to British and Dutch in colonies in India. Sent men to SA to obtain but failed. Finally Charles Ledger, an Australian, convinced an Indian, Manuel Incra, to collect seeds from a high-yielding tree. He did, was discovered, and killed. Ledger sent seeds to London which did not want them because a previous batch was low in quality. The Dutch bought one pound of seeds for the equivalent of $20. High quality, became basis of huge industry. By 1930 Dutch plantations produced 22 million pounds - 97% of world's quinine.

In 1940 Germans seized entire European repository when it captured Amsterdam. When Japanese conquered Indonesia in 1942, US & allies with quinine. Small plantation in Philippines soon fell, too. Last allied plane to leave carried 4 million seeds flown to Maryland to germinate and planted in Costa Rica.

Little hope could mature fast enough. More Americans died from malaria than fighting.

Botanist Raymond Fosberg was dispatched to the Andes to find bark. He collected 12.5 million pounds. Learned about biology of Cinchona but never found original high yielding species. Synthetics lacked efficacy, unpleasant side effects (nausea, diarrhea and yellowing of skin).

WWII stopped flow to Allied countries. Japanese invasion of Dutch East Indies in 1942 captures. Then in 1944 synthesized, but expensive.

Botanical Explorations: There are about 40 species of Cinchona, lots of varieties and produce varying amounts of active ingredients. They grow on the slopes of the Andes high in the rain forest. Use bark. In coffee family (Rubiaceae). Linnaeus named after Countess of Cinchon, wife of the Viceroy of Peru. Legend suggests that she has was miraculously cured in 1638 by the bark.

Physiological Activity: In 1820 isolated alkaloid quinine by French chemists M. Pelletier and Joseph Caventou.

Chemistry: Quinine active ingredient.

XII. Medicinal Plant Quickies.

1. Mexican yams (Dioscorea sp).

The tubers are collected and processed to extract diosgenin and steroidal materials. Processed to provide precursors for birth control pills and other steroids. Mimics the effect of progesterone in preventing ovulation.

2. Ginseng (Panax quinquefolia)—extremely important in Chinese medicine. Taproot used as a general tonic. Root human-like appearance. Perhaps responsible (*i.e.*, Doctrine of Signatures). Commands high price, collected to near extinction.
3. Rosy periwinkle (Cantharanthus roseus)—used to treat leukemia, Hodgkin's. Discovered from a healer's claims that it was useful against diabetes. Produces a variety of alkaloids including vinblastine and vincristine. Lily Co. discovered in screenings.

4. Ginkgo (Ginkgo biloba)—deciduous gymnosperm. treat senility, memory loss.
5. Echinacea-infections, boost immune system
6. St. John's Wort or Hypericum-depression
7. Saw palmetto-prostrate (not covered)
8. Cranberry-urinary tract disorders. (not covered)

XIII. Animals and Medicinal Plants. (not covered)

Humans weren't the first to use plants for medicine - other animals do, too. Zoopharmacognosy, first reported in 1987 by Eloy Rodriquez and Richard Wrangham. Wooly spider monkeys in Brazil eat fruits of the "Monkey Ear" plant to enhance fertility.

This plant has since been shown to be rich in the steroid stigmasterol. Bears chew the roots of Ligusticum porteri (Carrot Family) and smear it on their fur. Contains coumarins that act as flea and tick repellent. Chimps eat Aspilia and Vernonia (both Sunflower family) for infections and upset stomachs.

Commonly Used Medicinal Plants

The most common diseases during the middle ages were dysentery, epilepsy, influenza, diphtheria, scurvy, typhoid, smallpox, scabies, impetigo, leprosy, pneumonia, stroke, heart attack, scrofula (chronically swollen lymph nodes, later identified as a form of tuberculosis), St. Vitus' Dance (rheumatic chorea, a temporary disorder of the parts of the brain that control movement and coordination), and St. Anthony's Fire (ergotism, caused by ingesting toxic amounts of alkaloids produced by a fungus that infests rye - symptoms included gangrene with burning pain in the extremities, convulsions, hallucinations, and severe psychosis).

Plants listed in this section are those used most frequently to treat these and other illnesses. Quoted excerpts of treatments from medical texts were translated from Middle English.

Aloe: Greek physician Dioscorides recommended aloe externally for wounds, hemorrhoids, ulcers and hair loss. Pliny prescribed it internally as a laxative.

Angelica (Wild Celery): Angelica leaf necklaces were worn as protection against illness and witchcraft. Angelica was reputed to be the only herb witches never used and its presence in a woman's garden or cupboard was successfully used as a defense against charges of witchcraft. Gilbert Anglicus' Compendium of Medicine gives the following prescription for using angelica as a cough remedy: And if the cough is of sticky thick phlegm, give him a syrup made with horehound, the root of fennel, radish, wild celery and anise.

Anise: Hippocrates recommended anise to help clear mucus from the respiratory system. It was also recommended by other renowned physicians as a breath freshener, digestive aid, a cure for "hicket" (hiccups), headache, asthma, insomnia, nausea, lice and infant colic. Anise was so popular in medieval England as a spice, medicine and perfume that in 1305 Edward I placed a special tax on it to raise money to repair London Bridge.

Apple: Hildegard of Bingen prescribed raw apples as a tonic for healthy people and cooked apples as the first treatment for any sickness.

Balm (Melissa): Lemon balm and bee balm were prescribed for nervousness and anxiety in the form of Melissa water or Eau de Melisse. Recommended for treatment of insomnia, arthritis, headache, toothache, sores, digestive problems and cramps, balm was considered to be something of a cure-all. Greek physicians recommended applying balm leaves to wounds and added the herb to wine to treat a variety of illnesses. Pliny prescribed it to stop bleeding.

Basil: The ancient physicians disagreed on the merits of basil. Dioscorides and Galen warned that taking basil internally would cause insanity and the spontaneous generation of internal worms. Pliny used it to treat stomach ailments. Hildegard of Bingen used basil in a concoction that included powder from a vulture's beak to treat tumors.

Blackberry: Blackberry was also known as "goutberry" as its most popular use was as a treatment for gout. Leaves and bark were chewed for bleeding gums, leaves were applied to the skin to sooth burns and scalds. Blackberry syrup was recommended for treatment of dysentery.

Buckthorn : Buckthorn became popular around the 13th century and was primarily used to purge the body of "foul humors". Buckthorn bark seeped in water produced a powerful laxative. It was also recommended for jaundice, hemorrhoids, gout and arthritis.

Burdock : In the 14th century burdock leaves were used to treat leprosy. Hildegard of Bingen used it to treat cancerous tumours. Burdock root was also prescribed for fever, ringworm and skin infections.

Caraway : Caraway seeds were recommended for the treatment of indigestion, gas and infant colic. Gilbertus Anglicus prescribed the following decoction for a syrup to treat ailments of the lungs: Take barley water which has been strained, raisins, violets, jujube, seed of melon and gourd, wheat starch, licorice, black plums, fennel root, parsley, wild celery, anise, caraway, and make thereof a syrup. That is to say, seep all these in water until the virtue of them be in the water. Then strain it and add sugar or honey. And then set it over the fire to steep softly. Then take the white of four eggs and beat them well and add them. And always skim it until it is clear. Then take it down and strain it clean so that no dregs remain therein. Put it in a closed vessel.

Chamomile : Used to treat headaches, kidney, liver and bladder problems and as an aid for digestive upsets.

Cinnamon : Hildegard of Bingen recommended cinnamon to treat colds, flu, cancer and "inner decay and slime."

Coltsfoot : Used for treating coughs, wheezing, shortness of breath, fever and inflammation.

Comfrey : Boiling comfrey root in water produced a thick paste in which cloth was soaked and then wrapped around broken bones. Internally, comfrey was used for treating respiratory and gastrointestinal problems.

Dandelion : Dandelion was prescribed to treat colds, boils, ulcers, dental problems, itching, jaundice and gallstones.

Dill : Digestive aid and gas remedy. Also a cure for hiccups. From Gilbertus Anglicus' Compendium of Medicine this treatment for squinacy (quinsy):

But if a postem be of phlegm, after his blood-letting and his purging, make him a gargle of sap from a hazelnut tree, dill, poppy, either the water that bark from a nut or mulberry tree has been seeped in, or the juice of bittersweet, with dried honeysuckle leaves and aloe.

Elecampane : Prescribed to treat coughs, bronchitis, asthma and indigestion.

Fennel : The ancient physicians prescribed fennel to treat infant colic, as an appetite suppressant and recommended the seeds to nursing mothers to boost milk production. Pliny believed that fennel was a cure for eye problems, including blindness. Hildegard of Bingen recommended fennel for treating colds, heart ailments and to aid in good digestion and body odour. Folk healers mixed fennel with strong laxatives such as buckthorn to counteract intestinal cramps.

Fenugreek : Fenugreek seeds mixed with water was used as a salve to soothe inflamed or irritated tissue. Internally, it was used to treat fever and digestion and respiratory ailments. Gilbertus Anglicus considered a plaster using fenugreek (femigreke) in combination with a gargle made of other ingredients to be somewhat of a cure-all:

Good for every postem both within a man's body and without: Take the root of hollyhock and lily roots and seep them in water. Then crush them with fresh grease and butter and add meal of flax seed (linseed) and fenugreek and snails and crush them together. And give him a gargle of vinegar that barley has lain in and water that pomegranate or sumac or roses or oak galls or lentils have soaked in.

Garlic : Greek and Roman physicians recommended garlic for infections, wounds, cancer, leprosy, heart problems, colds, and epilepsy among many other ailments. In the middle ages the upper class shunned the use of garlic, but the peasantry viewed it as a preventative medicine and cure-all.

Horehound : First used in ancient Rome as an ingredient in poison antidotes lead medieval Europeans to believe horehound provided protection from wtiches' spells. Hildegard of Bingen considered it one of the best herbs for colds. Galen was the first to recommend horehound for coughs and respiratory problems.

Hyssop : Prescribed for use in a tea for coughs, wheezing and shortness of breath and in plasters and salves for chest decongestion. Hildegard of Bingen recommended a meal of chicken stewed in hyssop and wine as a treatment for depression.

Licorice : Hippocrates recommended licorice for cough, asthma and other respiratory diseases. Hildegard of Bingen prescribed it for stomach problems.

Mint : Spearmint was the original medicinal mint and was used to aid in digestion and the treatment of gout. In Gilbertus Anglicus' Compendium of Medicine the following treatment is recommended for "stinking of the mouth":

If there be no rotten flesh, let the mouth be washed with wine that birch or mint has been soaked in. And let the gums be well rubbed with a rough linen cloth until they bleed. And let him eat marjoram, mint and parsley till they be well chewed. And let him rub well his teeth with the herbs he chewed and also his gums.

Motherwort : Used to treat heart palpitations and depression; later to stimulate contractions during childbirth.

Myrrh : Myrrh was valued primarily as an oral treatment for bleeding gums, mouth ulcers and sore throat. It was also used as an expectorant for colds and congestion.

Oregano : Used as a digestive aid, arthritis treatment, expectorant for cough, colds and chest congestion.

Parsley : Galen prescribed parsley for epilepsy and as a diuretic to treat water retention. Hildegard of Bingen recommended parsley compresses for arthritis and parsley boiled in wine for chest and heart pain.

Pennyroyal (Fleabane) : Pliny first discovered that when rubbed on the skin or strewn, penyroyal repelled fleas. He also recommended it as a cough remedy and digestive aid. Taken with honey, pennyroyal was said to cleanse the lungs and clear the chest of "all gross and thick humours".

Roses : Hippocrates recommended rose flowers mixed with oil for diseases of the uterus. Hildegard of Bingen prescribed rose hip tea as the initial treatment for many complaints including headache, dizziness and cramps. For difficulty in swallowing, Gilbertus Anglicus recommended a syrup called "honey roset" which consisted of a pound of minced roses soaked in a pound of honey over a fire.

Rosemary : In 1235 Queen Elizabeth of Hungary became paralyzed. According to legend, a hermit soaked a pound of rosemary in a gallon of wine for several days then rubbed it on her limbs, curing her. Rosemary/wine combinations became known as Queen of Hungary's Water and were used externally to treat skin problems, gout, dandruff, and prevention of baldness.

Saffron : Rare in Europe until after the Crusades, by the 14th century saffron was recommended to treat jaundice, insomnia and cancer.

Sage : Sage was considered to be something of a cure-all. Pliny prescribed it for snakebite, epilepsy, intestinal worms and chest ailments. Dioscorides recommended using sage leaves as bandages for wounds. Gilbertus Anglicus recommends the following for aching eyes:

And if it (the ache of the eyes) comes of phlegm purge it as I told in the headache and in other sicknesses of the head. And if it be of melancholy, purge it. And afterward let him be stood over a stew five or seven times, that is made of wormwood, betony, fennel, sage, flowers of thyme, chamomile flowers, melilot flowers, hock, and wild celery. All these must be soaked in wine and water together, half wine and the other half water. And let him hold his eyes and his head over the stew. And afterward take a linen cloth or cotton and wet in the water. And annoint therewith his eyes.

St. John's Wort : Early physicians prescribed St. John's Wort taken internally with wine as a cure for poisonous snakebite and externally as a treatment for burns. Christians believed that St. John's wort repelled evil spirits and burned it in bonfires on St. John's Eve to purify the air, drive away evil spirits and ensure healthy crops.

Thyme : Thyme was used as a cough remedy, digestive aid and treatment for intestinal worms. Hildegard of Bingen favoured it for skin problems. Thyme was also recommended to those who suffered from depression; they were advised to sleep on thyme-stuffed pillows. Gilbertus Anglicus recommended the following involved treatment for a soft spleen:

For softness of the spleen, if it be of cold humours give him oximel (medicine made of two parts vinegar and one of honey) to defy the humours. Afterward give him iera pigra Galieni (a decoction made of valerian, cinnamon, saffron, camel hay, hazelwort, bark of cassia and balsa, violets, wormwood, roses, gourds and alloes among other spices) to purge the humours. After the third day treat with a bath of hot herbs such as oregano, mint, horehound, thyme, rosemary and such others. And the next day let him bleed under the ankle in the underside of the left foot. And make him hot plasters of rue, celandine, and nettles to consume the humours and lay to the spleen.

Valerian : Ancient physicians recommended valerian as a diuretic, antidote to poisons, for pain relief and as a decongestant. Hildegard of Bingen prescribed it as a tranquilizer and sleeping aid.

Vervain : In the middle ages healing herbs were called simples. Vervain was prescribed so often and for so many different ailments that it became known as "simpler's joy." It was recommended for fever, tumours, blood infections, toothache, and acne among many other ailments.

Yarrow : Used to treat inflammations, to stop bleeding, as a digestive aid, for pain relief and as a mild sedative.

Medicinal Plants as a Part of Culture

It is evident that the Indian people have a tremendous passion for medicinal plants and use them for a wide range of health related applications from a common cold to memory improvement and treatment of poisonous snake bites to a cure for muscular distrophy and the enhancement of body's general immunity. In the oral traditions local communities in every ecosystem from the trans himalayas down to the coastal plains have discovered the medical uses of thousands of plants found locally in their ecosystem. India has one of the richest plant medical culture in the world. It is a culture that is of tremendous contemporary relevance because it can on one hand ensure health security to millions of people and on the other hand it can provide new and safe herbal drugs to the entire world. There are estimated to be around 25000 effective plant based formulations are available in the indigenous medical texts formulations used in folk medicine and known to rural communities all over India and around 10000 designed.

Distribution

Macro analysis of the distribution of medicinal plants show that they are distributed across diverse habitats and landscape elements. Around 70% of India's medicinal plants are found in tropical areas mostly in the various forest types spread across the Western and Eastern ghats, the Vindhyas, Chotta Nagpur plateau, Aravalis & Himalayas. Although less than 30% of the medicinal plants are found in the temperate and alpine areas and higher altitudes they include species of high medicinal value. Macro studies show that a larger percentage of the known medicinal plant occur in the dry and moist deciduous vegetation as compared to the evergreen or temperate habitats.

Analysis of habits of medicinal plants indicate that they are distributed across various habitats. One third are trees and an equal portion shrubs and the remaining one third herbs, grasses and climbers. A very small proportion of the medicinal plants are lower plants like lichens, ferns algae, etc. Majority of the medicinal plant are higher flowering plants.

Distribution of Medicinal Plants by Habits

Of the 386 families and 2200 genera in which medicinal plants are recorded, the families Asteraceae. Euphorbiacae. Laminaceae, Fabaceae, Rubiaceae., Poaceae, Acanthaceae, Rosaceae and Apiaceae share the larger proportion of medicinal plant species with the highest number of species (419) falling under Asteraceae.

About 90% of medicinal plant used by the industries are collected from the wild. While over 800 species are used in production by industry, less than 20 species of plants are under commercial cultivation. Over 70% of the plant collections involve destructive harvesting because of the use of parts like roots, bark, wood, stem and the whole plant in case of herbs. This poses a definite threat to the genetic stocks and to the diversity of medicinal plants if biodiversity is not sustainably used.

Conservation and Development of Medicinal Plants

Medicinal plants continue to be an important therapeutic aid for alleviating ailments of humankind. Search for eternal health and longevity and to seek remedy to relieve pain and discomfort prompted the early man to explore his immediate natural surrounding and tried many plants, animal products and minerals and developed a variety of therapeutic agents. Over millenia that followed the effective agents amongst them were selected by the process of trial, error, empirical reasoning and even by experimentation. These efforts have gone in history by the name discovery of `medicine'.

In many eastern cultures such as those of India, China and the Arab/Persian world this experience was systematically recorded and incorporated into regular system of medicine that refined and developed and became a part of the Materia Medica of these countries. The ancient civilization of India, China, Greece, Arab and other countries of the world developed their systems of medicine independent of each other but all of them were predominantly plant based.

But the theoretical foundation and the insights and indepth understanding on the practice of medicine that we find in Ayurveda is much superior among organized ancient systems of medicine. From history we learn that in the ancient times India was known as a place of rich natural resources, knowledge, wisdom and scholarship. People from other countries of the world as China, Cambodia, Indonesia and Baghdad used to come to the ancient universities of India like Takshila (700 BC) and Nalanda (500 BC) to learn health sciences of India, particularly `Ayurveda'. It is perhaps the oldest (6000 BC) among the organized traditional medicine. It has gone through several stages of development in its long history. It spread with Vedic, Hindu and the Buddhist cultures and reached as far as Indonesia in the east and to the west it influenced the ancient Greek who developed a similar form of medicine.

All Systems of Medicine in India functions through two social streams: Folk Stream: Comprising mostly the oral traditions practiced by the rural villages. The carriers of these traditions are millions of housewives, thousands of traditional birth attendants, bone setters, village practitioners skilled in accupressure, eye treatments, treatment of snake bites and the traditional village physicians/herbal healers, the vaidyas' or the tribal physicians.

This stream of inherited traditions are together known as Local Health Traditions (LHT). LHT represent an autonomous community supported health management system which efficiently and effectively manage the primary health care of the Indian rural mass. LHT is still alive and runs parallel to the state supported modern health care system; but its full potential is still not fully utilized and also that the great service it is rendering to the rural people go largely unnoticed because of the dominant western medicine.

Classical stream: At the second level of traditional health care system is the scientific or classical systems of medicine. This comprises of the codified and organized medicinal wisdom with sophisticated theoretical foundations and philosophical explanations expressed in classical texts like `Charka Samhita', `Sushruta samhita', 'Bhela samhita', and hundreds of other treatises including some in the regional languages covering treaties of all branches of medicine and surgery. Systems like Ayurveda, Siddha, Unani, Amchi and Tibetan, etc. are expressions of the same. Ayurveda was taught in the ancient universities in India and evolved, developed and flourished mostly among the urban centres and thus used to be a refined system of medicine.

Revival of Traditional Medicine

Today we find a renewed interest in traditional medicine. During the past decade there have been an ever increasing demand especially from developed countries for more and more drugs from plant sources. This revival of interest in plant derived drugs is mainly due to the current widespread belief that `green medicine' is safe and more dependable than the costly synthetic drug many of which have adverse side effects. This resurgence of interest in the plant based drugs have necessitated an increased demand of medicinal plants leading to over-exploitation, unsustainable harvesting and finally to the virtual decimation of several valuable plant species in the wild.

Moreover, the habitat degradation due to increased human activities (human settlements, agriculture and other developmental programmes), illegal trade in rare and endangered medicinal plants, and loss of regeneration potential of the degraded forests have further accelerated the current rate of extinction of plants particularly the medicinal plants.

Medicinal Plants Wealth of India

India is rich in medicinal plant diversity. All known types of agroclimatic, ecologic and edaphis conditions are met within India. The biogeographic position of India is so unique that all known types of ecosystems ranging from coldest place like the Nubra Valley with - 570 C, dry cold deserts of Ladakh, temperate and Alpine and subtropical regions of the North-West and trans-Himalayas, rain forests with the world's highest rainfall in Cheerapunji in Meghalaya, wet evergreen humid tropics of Western Ghats, arid and semi-arid conditions of Peninsular India, dry desert conditions of Rajasthan and Gujarat to the tidal mangroves of the Sunderban.

India is rich in all the three levels of biodiversity-such as species diversity, genetic diversity and habitat diversity. There are about 426 biomes representing different habitat diversity that gave rise to one of the richest centres in the world for plant genetic resources. The total number of flowering plant species although only 17,000, the intraspecific variability found in them make it one of the highest in the world. Out of 17,000 plants, the classic systems of medicines like Ayurveda, Siddha and Unani make use of only about 2000 plants in various formulations.

The classical traditions were prevalent in the past particularly in the urban elite society. The rural people who constitute 70 to 75% of the Indian populations live in about

5,76,000 villages located in different agroclimatic conditions. The village people have their own diverse systems of health management. While most of the common ailments were managed in the house by home remedies which included many species and condiments like pepper, ginger, turmeric, coriander, cumins, tamarind, fenagree, tulsi, etc., more complicated cases were attended by the traditional physicians who use a large number of plants from the ambient vegetations and some products of animal or mineral origin to deal with the local diseases and ailments.

These are indeed community managed systems independent of official or government system and are generally known as Local Health Tradition (LHT). The traditional village physicians of India are using about 4500 to 5000 species of plants for medicinal purpose. There is however no systematic, inventory and documentation about the folk remedies of India. There is urgent need to document this fast disappearing precious knowledge system. The oral traditions of the villagers use about 5000 plant for medicinal purposes. India is also inhabited by a large number of tribal communities who also posses a precious and unique knowledge about the use of wild plants for treating human ailments.

A survey conducted by the All India Coordinated Research Project on Ethnobiology (AICRPE) during the last decade recorded over 8000 species of wild plants used by the tribals and other traditional communities in India for treating various health problems. Some interesting observations made in the study is the use of the same species found in different regions for the same ailments while some other species are used differentially.

Strategies & Priorities

The world conservation strategy (IUCN, UNEP & WWF, 1980) defines conservations as "the management of human use of the biodiversity so that it may yield the greatest sustainable benefit to present generation while maintaining its potential to meet the needs and aspirations of future generations". The above definition invokes two complementary components "conservation" and "sustainability". The primary goals of biodiversity conservation as envisaged in the World Conservation Strategy can be summarised as follows:

1. Maintenance of essential ecological processes and life support systems on which human survival and economic activities depend,
2. Preservation of species and genetic diversity and
3. Sustainable use of species and ecosystems which support millions of rural communities as well as major industries.

Medicinal plants are potential renewable natural resources. Therefore, the conservation and sustainable utilisation of medicinal plants must necessarily involve a long term, integrated, scientifically oriented action programme. This should involve the pertinent aspects of protection, preservation, maintenance, exploitation, conservation and sustainable utilization. A holistic and systematic approach envisaging interaction between social, economic and ecological systems will be a more desirable one. The most widely accepted scientific technologies of biodiversity conservation are the in-situ and ex-situ methods.

In-situ Conservation

In has been well established that the best and cost-effective way of protecting the existing biological and genetic diversity is the 'in-situ' or on the site conservation wherein a wild species or stock of a biological community is protected and preserved in its natural habitat. The prospect of such a 'ecocentric', rather than a species centred approach is that it should prevent species from becoming endangered by human activities and reduce the need for human intervention to prevent premature extinctions. Establishment of biosphere reserves, national parks, wild life sanctuaries, sacred groves and other protected areas forms examples of 'in-situ' methods of conservation.

The idea of establishing protected area network has taken a central place in all policy decision process related to biodiversity conservation at national, international and global level.

In India 4.5% of its total geographical area constitute protected area network, comprising 8 designated biospheres, 87, national parks, 447 wild life sanctuaries.

This network encompasses various biogeographic zones and biomes rich in biotic diversity, including medicinal and aromatic plants. In addition to these there area number of sacred groves in different parts of the country particularly in South, West and Eastern parts which are also active centres on in-situ conservation of medicinal plants. Such conservation area network can attribute significantly towards the conservation and sustainable management of biological resources of our country.

However, experiences have amply demonstrated that in a densely populated developing country like India, where a sizeable population are living in close proximity to forests, declaring protected areas will not entirely be sufficient to ensure conservation on the fast eroding biological diversity. The success of any conservation programme vests solely on the efficient management of protected areas.

The involvement of local communities in conservation activities has now been increasingly realised. A people nature-oriented approach thus become highly imperative. This will help to generate a sense of responsibility among the local people about the values of biodiversity and the need to use it sustainably for their own prosperity and the maintenance of ecosystem resilience.

In-situ conservation of medicinal plants in India can be accomplished through the active support and participation of people who dwell in or near and around the protected forest areas. Involving the local mass in all phases of conservation programmes, such as planning, policy-decision process, implementation etc will be a significant component in achieving efficient management and utilization of medicinal plant resources. A few such in-situ conservation areas have been marked and declared as medicinal plant in-situ conservation areas on the forests of three Southern States of Kerala, Tamil Nadu and Karnataka by the joint efforts of the forest departments of these States and FRLHT, Bangalore.

Ex-situ Conservation

Conservation of medicinal plants can be accomplished by the ex-situ *i.e.* outside natural habitat by cultivating and maintaining plants in botanic gardens parks, other suitable sites, and through long term preservation of plant propagules in gene banks (seed bank, pollen bank, DNA libraries, etc.) and in plant tissue culture repositories and by cryopreservation).

Botanical gardens can play a key role in ex-situ conservation of plants, especially those facing imminent threat of extinction. Several gardens in the world are specialised in cultivation and study of medicinal plants, while some contain a special medicinal plant garden or harbour special collection of medicinal plants.

India has a network of about 140 botanical gardens which include 33 botanical gardens attached to 33 universities botany departments. But hardly 30 botanical gardens have any active programme on conservation. Tropical Botanical Gardens & Research Institute (TGBRI), located in a degraded forest region of Western Ghat mountains in Kerala has an excellent example in ex-situ conservation of plant diversity in India. The field gene bank programme launched by TBGRI from 1992-1999 is now well acclaimed as a very effective method of conservation of medicinal and aromatic plant genetic resources. This field gene bank of medicinal and aromatic plants at TBGRI, Thiruvananthapuram is essentially a blend of the ex-situ and in-situ situations.

Field Gene Bank of Medicinal Plants: The concept of establishing field gene banks of plants provide ample options for long term preservation of the genetic variability (inter-specific) of species. Field gene banks are better established in a degraded forests where efforts could be made to reforest/ restock the missing species complexes, trees, shrubs, herbs, climber etc. It is indeed a recreation of a forest or rather simulation of a typical forest. Before attempting to establish such a field gene bank it is essential to have a clear understanding of the natural ecosystem such as the spatial distribution, pattern of association *i.e.*, structure and functional dynamics of the species in question. After undertaking a in depth study on the natural distribution pattern of the medicinal plants and the associated floristic elements - including their micro-ecological niche, a well planned action programme of recreating the same in a degraded forest area or place close to the species found in nature can be attempted. TBGRI has accomplished this task of simulating the nature while establishing the field gene bank of medicinal and aromatic plants under the G-15-GBMAP sponsored by DBT, Government of India. TBGRI experience now provide ample opportunity to repeat the same elsewhere in the country.

Identification of the keystone species and umbrella species are very important in this methods. After planting the keystone and umbrella species, other species complex which include the medicinal aromatic plants in question have to be introduced. The sampling and selection of samples for introduction have to be highly knowledge and science intensive. To capture the maximum possible genetic diversity of the target species it is extremely important to collect all valuable information such as morphological variants, chemical variants or genetic variants or chemical screening of the population of the targeted species by using the latest methods and tools.

The field gene bank of TBGRI has covered 30,000 accessions of 250 medicinal and aromatic plant species which include 100 endemic, rare and endangered medicinal and aromatic plants of the tropical region of India. A broad spectrum of the genetic diversity of these species were captured and introduced in this gene bank which covered morphotypes, cytotypes and chemotype and the number of samples from each species varied from 50-1000 plants.

Schemes of Different Agencies

National Parks and Sanctuaries

The National Parks and Wildlife Sanctuaries are protected areas encompassing the Biological Diversity in its pristine condition. At present there are 87 National Parks and 447 Wildlife Sanctuaries extending over an area of about 1.5 lakh sq. Km, which is more than 4.5% of the genographical area of the country. The National Parks stretch over 34,819 Sq. Km while the Sanctuaries cover an area of 1,15,903 Sq. Km.

A centrally sponsored scheme for the development of National Parks and Sanctuaries is in operation since VI Plan period. The main objective of the scheme is to support protection and conservation measures in these areas with a view to mitigate any adverse impact of biotic pressure and allowing the areas to rejuvenate through habitat manipulation and infrastructure development. During the VIII Plan Rs. 49.5 crores have been spent under this scheme and for IX Plan the outlay is Rs. 110 crores. Assistance is also provided for eco-development programmes around National Parks and Sanctuaries in order to achieve a ecologically sustainable economic development.

These protected areas harbour large varieties of medicinal plants. In-situ conservation programmes for medicinal plants in the National Parks and Sanctuaries could be taken up through Chief Wild Life Wardens. The programme needs to be in consonance with the objectives of the national parks and Sanctuaries.

Ethnobiological Studies

An All India Coordinated Research Project of Ethnobiology (AICRPE) under the Man and Biosphere was funded by the Ministry of Environment and Forests. The programme was executed by Tropical Botanical Garden Research Institute, Thiruvananthapuram and in association with other institutions such as Central Drug Research Institute (CDRI), Lucknow, Ethnobiology and Plant Systematic Laboratory, Garhwal, Botanical Survey of India, International Institute of Ayurveda, Coimbatore, etc. The first phase of the programme was completed in 6 years and was extended into the second phase. The study has covered about 80% of the tribal areas.

The data recorded on Indian ethnobiology is invaluable giving a status on the tribal communities along with the information on the ethnobiological inventorisation and their documentation. The study provides information on the wild plants used by the tribal communities as food, fodder etc., which also includes a large number of medicinal plants. The study reveals the sustained usage of the local resources and the natural system of conservation. However, this natural balance is being disturbed due to the intervention by other communities exploiting the medicinal plant resources. Data obtained from this study needs to be used in the process of planning and programme to conserve the rich biodiversity in our country. The focus on the medicinal plants resources and further investigation in these areas may lead to concrete programme for the conservation of medicinal plants.

Sacred Groves

There is no separate scheme for the Conservation or restoration of sacred groves under National Afforestation and Eco-development Board (NAEB). Documentation of the Sacred Groves have been carried out by the Regional Centres of the NAEB under the scheme to "Support to Regional Centres". There are seven regional centres and their activities include helping the State/UT Forest Departments and Forest Development Corporation in formulation of projects, conduct study research and educational programmes for the protection, development and improvement of forest area and the degraded forest areas.

Some Regional Centres have taken up the studies on the Sacred Groves under the forest protection and documentation. Such studies are proposed in the Annual Work Programme to the NAEB. The cost of the documents prepared are fixed on a case by case basis. The Work done so far included.

Studies have also been conducted by NGOs and research organisations to evaluate the status of sacred groves. The C.P.R Environmental Education Centre, Chennai is one of such an autonomous Centre of excellence of the Ministry of Environment & Forests. They have published books on the Sacred Trees of Tamil Nadu and Ecological Traditions of Tamil Nadu. A UNESCO study on the sacred groves of India provides a comprehensive picture of these groves along with their status. Some of the large groves and community associated with them have been presented as case studies.

However, a systematic nationwide survey of sacred groves have not been undertaken to account for the status of these groves in terms of the conservation of biological diversity and the traditional particular of the community. The most important of all is the legal status and ownership of the grove. The changing pattern of life styles and religious beliefs are also responsible for the deteriorating conditions of some of the groves.

NAEB's Scheme on Non-Timber Forest Produce including Medicinal Plants

Forest areas are the main source of medicinal plants, particularly the undisturbed natural forests. The medicinal plants from forests form an important component of the Minor Forest Produce, otherwise known as Non-Timber Forest Produce. Extraction of such produce including the medicinal plants from these areas is a traditional right of the local communities/tribals.

The National Afforestation and Eco-development Board (NAEB) has a mandate of promoting afforestation, tree planting, ecological restoration and eco-development activities in the country. Special attention is given to the regeneration of degraded forest areas and lands adjoining forest areas, national parks, sanctuaries and other protected areas as well the ecologically fragile areas like the Western Himalayas, Aravallis, Western Ghats etc.

A Centrally Sponsored Scheme of Minor Forest Produce was started in 1988-89 (Seventh Plan). The scheme provides 100% central assistance to the States and included following activities:

a. Mixed plantation of bamboo with fruit bearing species (harra, imli, mahua, char, aam etc. and oilseed bearing trees;
b. Plantation of tendu bushes under light canopy of trees;
c. Plantation of cane;
d. Cultivation of medicinal plants like Rauwolfia spp, Dioscorea spp to augment the rising demand for plant-based drugs and to offest the scarcity because of unscientific exploitation;
e. Cultivation of rosha grass/lemon grass.

During the Ninth Five Year Plan, the scheme is being operated in 25 States. The financial allocation is Rs. 80.50 crores. The grant released during 1997-98 and 1998-99 was Rs. 7.50 crores and Rs. 10.00 crores respectively. The outlay for 1999-2000 is Rs. 12 crores.

The main objectives of the scheme are:

i. Conservation and improvement of the non-timber forest produce, including medicinal plants;

ii. Increasing the production of and replenishing the stock of non-timber forest produce and medicinal plants; and

iii. Providing additional income to the tribals and the rural poor living in and around forests.

Forest Departments and Forest Development Corporation in States and Union Territories are the nodal agencies for implementation of the scheme. Project areas are confined mainly to recorded forest land.

JFM is a central and integral part of all plantation projects. The project authorities are being given adequate leverage by way of "entry-point activites" and requisite funds for building awareness amongst communities. In the selection of the project sites, gram panchayats or other village bodies are to be associated in project preparation, implementation and usufruct sharing in consonance with provisions of the Forest (Conservation) Act, 1980 and the guidelines issued in June, 1990.

UNDP-CCP I Assisted Sub-Programme on "Medicinal Plants Conservation and Sustaianble Utilisation"

A UNDP Country Cooperation Programme assisted Sub-programme on "Medicinal Plants Conservation and Sustainable Utilisation" has been approved and initiated in December, 1999. Foundation for Revitalization of Local Health Traditions (FRLHT), Bangalore has been designated as the coordinating agency. This is a demonstration project to replicate the activities being carried out in the three Southern States of Karnataka, Kerala and Tamil Nadu and in the States of Andhra Pradesh and Maharashtra. The executing agencies in Andhra Pradesh is Environmental Protection Training Research Institute

(EPTRI), Hyderabad and Rural Communes (RC), Mumbai in Maharashtra. The State Forest Department are the key players in the activities and would be responsible for providing the forest land for the in-situ conservation activities envisaged in the programme.

The activities include survey and inventorisation of medicinal plants in the selected areas in the State of Andhra Pradesh and Maharashtra. Identification of the sites for In-situ conservation. It would also include setting up of 8 Medicinal Plants Conservation Areas (MPCAs) in each of these states. The MPCAs thus set up would be repositories of the genetic material and the area would be demarcated as "no harvest zones". One of the important features is the threat assessment of the medicinal plant species by conducting "Rapid Threat Assessment" using IUCN methodology.

The programme comprises of extensive field visits and preparing herbarium sheets. The community programmes envisaged under this project would provide an opportunity for interaction and exchange of views among the different communities. Extensive training programme is also envisaged to train different section of the community, the forest officersf and other field staff.

GEF Small Grants Programme

The United Nations Development Programme (UNDP) operates the Small Grants Programme on behalf of Global Environmental Facility (GEF). This provides support for small-scale community based activities which contribute to the four GEF thematic areas namely Bio-Diversity, Climate Change, Ozone layer depletion and International Waters. The SGP in India took off towards 1995 and the theme areas include Biodiversity and Climate Change. The GEF-SGP in India has been structured to operate in a decentralised manner with a National Co-ordinator based within the National Host Institution (NHI) which is Development Alternatives. A National Selection Committee (NSC) with members representing GOI, UNDP, research and voluntary organisations is responsible for overall coordination and approval of the projects.

The first phase of the GEF-SGP was set up with an initial outlay of US$ 300,000 to provide assistance to each individual project. Twenty Four projects were approved in 1995 and 1997 (20 on Biodiversity and 4 on Climate Change covering 12 States). The objectives of the programme include promoting innovative local response, capacity building, community based initiatives especially rural and tribal, create public awareness and strengthen NGOs.

The Phase-II of GEF-SGP was initiated in 1998 and the project were approved in the first meeting of the NSC held in March 1999. A sum of US$ 700,000 are made available and a number of projects on medicinal plants were considered in the meetings of NSC held. There are 11 projects on medicinal plants sanctioned under this scheme in the States of Assam, Gujarat, Himachal Pradesh, Kerala, Meghalaya, Nagaland, Rajasthan and Uttar Pradesh. These are being executed by grass root NGOs.

Future Strategies to be Adopted: For sustainable and equitable development of medicinal plant the various organisations of Ministry of Environment and Forests may adopt following strategies:-

Cultivation of Medicinal Plants

Given the demands of the market for a continuous and uniform supply of raw materials, and the increasing depletion of the forest resource base, expanding the number of medicinal plants in cultivation appears to be an important strategy for research and development. However, according to one estimate, of more than 400 plant species used for production of medicines by Indian Industry, less than 20 are currently under the cultivation in the country.

The potential returns to the farmer from cultivation of medicinal plants is reported to be quite high. A 1995 study suggested that the cultivation of certain high altitude Himalayan herbs could yield products priced anywhere between Rs. 7,150 to 55,000 per hectare although it is not clear at which point in the marketing chain these prices are paid (Nautiyal 1995). What is clear however is that although estimates of returns vary widely, medicinal plants can be valuable crops. Rao and Saxena (1994) reported average annual (per hectare) income of Rs. 120,000 through mixed cropping of high altitude medicinal herbs. High altitude medicinal tend to command higher prices but those of lower altitudes are still significant. Data for some low-altitude crops from the Amarkantak region of Madhya Pradesh show economic returns for four profitable species. Cultivation is clearly a sustainable alternative to collection of medicinal plants from the wild.

Most of the produce of cultivated medicinal and aromatic plants is exported as crude drugs *e.g.* Psyllium, senna leaves, opium poppy and Asgand. Unfortunately, however, due to emphasis being placed on important cash crops, as well as the fact that the majority of the cultivated species are not indigenous to India, most cultivation efforts are not alleviating the pressure being exerted on the natural resource base.

Nevertheless, a number of techniques have been developed to increase the quality and yield of many of the cultivated species. It is estimated that Indian public sector research institutions have developed standardized practices for the propagation and agronomy of a total of about 40 species.

Much of the research progress to date has resulted from the decision of the Indian Council for Agricultural Research (ICAR) to establish an All-India Coordinated Research Project on Medicinal and Aromatic Plants(AICRPMAP), in 1972, under the auspices of the National Bureau of Plant Genetic Resources (NBPGR). Efforts have mainly focused on the development of agro-technology techniques, including propagation methods for medicinal and aromatic plants. Aromatic plants have however tended to receive more attention, perhaps because their market values are in general more widely known.

ICAR works through a network of research stations, including the National Research Centre for Medicinal and Aromatic Plants located in Anand, Gujarat, which specializes in domestication, and has created structural links between the NBPGR and its Plant Breeding Division in order to develop improved varieties of some of the medicinal plant species used in allopathic preparations.

Another major national public research organisation, the Council for Scientific and Industrial Research (CSIR), has also played a significant role with regard to cultivation of medicinal plants, through its creation of (CIMAP), the Central Institute of Medicinal and Aromatic Plants, in Lucknow. CIMAP is now an eminent institution in India focusing on agro-technology as well as basic studies; improvement and enhancement of the resource base, and chemistry and related research regarding product development from plants.

In connection with the two major research efforts described above, the Central Government initiated a five year programme (1992-1997) implemented by the Ministry of Agriculture to accelerate research and development of medicinal plants. With the support of 16 state agricultural universities, state horticulture and agriculture departments, regional research laboratories and the International Crop Research Institute for the Semi-Arid Tropics (ICRISAT), the GOI is establishing herbal gardens, nursery centres and demonstration seed production centres nationwide.

Ministry of Health & Family Welfare (Department of ISM&H) started a "central scheme for development and cultivation of medicinal plants" in the year 1990-91 to encourage development of agrotechnique for important species through Govt./semi-government organisations having expertise and infrastructure for this work. The scheme is expected to initiate studies on harvesting, drying, and storage of medicinal plants.

Private companies have also started to invest in the cultivation of medicinal plants, since they face difficulties with regard to increasing supply gaps as well as in some cases adulterated materials from the wild. One such company, the Arya Vaidya Sala, in Kottakal, Kerala, in addition to maintaining two large herbal gardens, has also undertaken research on the propagation of 10 species, the demand for which currently outstrips supply, or may soon do so.

Research and Development of Medicinal Plants

In order to fully convert the potential of our medicinal plants into economic wealth, a very active R&D programme is essential. The R & D has to cover all aspects relating to the species from collection to utilisation. For convenience we may categorise medicinal species into : (a) those which are of proven medicinal value as per scientific parameters, (b) those on which sufficient leads are available, and (c) those on which much work is required to be done.

Research investigations need to concentrate on the first two categories on the following aspects:-

- Evolving and optimising the most appropriate technologies for conservation, especially for endangered or endemic specie and molecular methods for characterisation.
- Detailed studies on life cycle and breeding behaviour, taxonomy, seed biology
- Population and habitat viability studies
- Optimising appropriate methods for Post Harvest handling, processing and storage.
- Investigation on quality control standardization and shelf life of raw materials and finished products.

The search for new drugs of plant origin has yielded fruitful result in the past. Today it is possible to use molecular techniques for detection of genetic variability and tagging desired traits as well as culling out duplicates in accessions. The availability of high throughout screen has made the possibility of converting 'hits' into lead compounds in comparatively short time. Drug development from plant sources using gene/molecular techniques is becoming increasingly important.

Drug Development from New Molecules/Genes

In terms of a modern research endeavour, drug development from plants must necessarily imply a multi-displinary approach. Recent computerised studies of ethnomedical information, albeit in specialised areas of biological activity, have nevertheless confirmed that plants are a reservoir of chemical agents with therapeutic potential. What has been hitherto missed is the collation of data gathered in the trial-and-error is a prolonged clinical trial.

This information includes:

a. Ethnomedical particulars on cultivation, gathering and preparation of plant material for dosage.
b. The role of accompanying plants frequently used in multicomponent traditional preparations.
c. Recommended dosage regiments and contra-indications of certain foods.

In addition, it would be wise, in any research effort, to investigate the theories and concepts of the major systems of traditional medicine, as these cannot always be exactly interpreted in terms of modern concepts.

In general, natural products that have come into modern medicine are the result of an approach to drug development adopted over the past fifty years or more. The goal has been to find new chemical structures that have a novel biological activity. The alternative approach of finding plant derived therapeutic agents as extracts that could be standardised and formulated, has not received attention. The emphasis of R&D should be on the following:

- Development of technology for bulk production of medicinal products;
- Development of quality control standards for the starting materials as well as for the finished products;
- Development of new formulations and dosage forms specially suited to the prevailing climatic conditions and adapted to locally available raw materials;
- Assimilation of acquired technology and its continuous improvement to make the products competitive;
- Bioequivalence, bioavailability and pharmacokinetic studies on the dosage forms developed;
- Search of new plant sources for known drug and for new drugs from locally available plants.

Given the situation, production of standardized plant fraction should have priority over that of pure active substance, because of the simple technology needed and hence lower cost of the product, provided, of course, the technological testing indicates that the product is safe. It would be advisable to find out the chemical composition of the composite fraction and pharmacological action of each constituent to ensure that they are safe and compatible with each other.

In view of the high capital and recurring costs of R & D, collaboration among developing countries and between developed and developing countries is advisable. Keeping in view the national priority the target disease is selected and the plants on the formulation is evaluated clinically using current protocols/criteria. Studies on analytical methods, details chemistry, pharmacology along with toxicity and safety aspects are required. A multidisciplinary approach to drug development from medicinal plants used in traditional medicine was tried out in several technical assistance programmes by UNIDO beginning in the mid-1970s.

- Economic mapping of the spontaneous flora.
- Selection and authentication of plant species.
- Collation of ethnomedical and ethnobotanical data.
- Trial popagation to develop high yielding varieties.
- Medium scale plant propagation.
- Chemical studies on plant constituents
- Analytical studies on quantitative assessment of major constituents.
- Pharmacological and toxicological studies
- Pilot plant scale processing of plant extracts.
- Standardisation of extracts.
- Formulation studies on extracts into dosage forms.
- Toxicity studies on formulations
- Analytical studies on formulated products

UNIDO's technical Assistance Programme envisaged that if a successful candidate plant was identified, then the large-scale plant cultivation was to be implemented with FAO and the clinical assessment of the drug be conducted with WHO participation. Success was recorded in a number of instances and the programme introduced the concept of goal-oriented research.

Ethnobotanical Approach to Drug Discovery

For pharmaceuticals ranging from digitalis to vincristine the ethnobotanical approach to drug discovery has proved successful. The advent of high-throughput, mechanism-based in vitro bioassays coupled with candidate plants derived from painstaking enthnopharmacological research has resulted in the discovery of new pharmaceuticals such as prostratin, a drug candidate for treatment of human immunodeficiency virus, as well as a variety of novel anti-inflammatory compounds. Gastro-intestinal maladies, inflammation, skin infections and certain viral diseases are likely to be of high saliency to indigenous healers, whereas diseases such as cancer and cardiovascular illness are unlikely to be easily diagnosed by indigenous peoples.

Yet indigenous remedies may indicate pharmacological activity for maladies such as schizophrenia, for which the biochemical mechanisms have yet to be discovered. Ethnopharmacological information can be used to provide three levels of resolution in the search for new drugs: (1) as a general indicator of non-specific bioactivity suitable for a panel of broad screens: (2) as an indicator of specific bioactivity suitable for particular high-resolution bioassays: (3) as an indicator of pharmacological activity for which mechanism-based bioassays have yet to be developed.

Historically, ethnobotanical leads have resulted in three different types of drug discovery: (1) unmodified natural plant products where ethnomedical use suggested clinical efficacy (e.g digitalis); (2) unmodified natural products of which the therapeutic efficacy was only remotely suggested by indigenous plant use (e.g vincristine); and (3) modified natural or synthetic substances based on a natural product used in folk medicine (e.g aspirin).

The NAPRALERT database developed by Farnsworth is especially through, with systematic searches dating back to 1900, on natural products in the areas of cancer (chemotherapy, chemoprevention, carcinogenesis), fertility regulation (both male and female), diabetes, malaria and other parasitic diseases, viral diseases, sugar substitutes, molluscicides and anti-HIV agents. As an exercise to demonstrate the power of computer analysis, selected 10 diseases searched NAPRALERT for species that had both ethnomedical information and in vitro and/or in vivo experimental data supporting the ethnomedical claims.

Bioengineering of Medicinal Plants

Pharmaceutical importance/therapeutic value of medicinal plants is due to specific constituents/combination of secondary metabolites present in them. Changes in the proportion of secondary metabolites are often required for the improvement of therapeutic values of medicinal plants. For example, increase in the artemisinin content of Artemisia annua in proportion to its immediate precursors and other terpenes is required to make the production of antimalarials from this plant more economically.

The biosynthetic pathways for the biologically active chemical compounds in medicinal plants are usually complex and high branches. Genetic manipulations can help increase/decrease the contents of specific compounds in medicinal plants. Detailed understanding of these pathways will be a prerequisite for the identification, cloning and genetic engineering of the concerned structural and regulatory genes. These genetic techniques will also help develop designer medicinal plants. For example it will be possible to produce medicinal plants that will help raise the immunity towards infectious diseases in the use of such plants.

In Vitro Propagation Techniques

The biotechnological tools are important to select, multiply and conserve the critical genotypes of medicinal plants by adopting techniques such as micropropagation, creation of somacional varations and genetic transformations. Biotechnological tools can also be harnessed for production of secondary metabolites using plants as bioreactors.

In vitro propagation involves cell culture systems of a range of ex-plant tissues and mostly micropropagation is achieved from organised tissues by multiplication of meristems and auxillary buds. In many cases it provides an opportunity to maintain type-to type plant species and the propagation system can produce a large number of plants from a single clone. Plant regeneration from shoot and stem meristems has yielded encouraging results in medicinal plants like Catharanthus roseus, Cinchona ledgeriana and Digitalis spp.

The production of tropane alkaloids by hairy root culture has been resorted in several medicinal plants like Atropa, Datura and Hyoscyamus. Plant cell suspension culture is the selection of variant cell lines for the genetic improvement of plants. High secondary product yields in plant cell cultures of medicinal plants like Catharanthus roseus, Coleus blumei, Coptis japonica and Panax ginseng have been reported. Cryopreservation has been used successfully to store a range of tissue types, including meristems, anthers/pollens, embryos, calli and even protoplasts. Cryopreservation is already reported for many medicinal plants like Rauvolfia serpentina, Datura spp., Atropa, Hyoscyamus spp. etc. Protoplast fusion or somatic hybridization has been used to bypass the sexual process.

The objective is to transfer important genes which can not be transferred through sexual means due to the operation of incompatibility systems. Somatic hybrids between Atropa belladona and Datura innoxia were reported which showed higher amounts of tropane alkaloids. Biotransformation of psychotrine cephaeline to emetine production from cell cultures of Ipecac needs to be shown economically viable when compared with synthetic process of production of emetine.

Plant cell culture is of ımportance of improvement of medicinal plants. Complete plants have been regenerated from callus cultures, excised anthers and isolated protoplasts of many medicinal and aromatic plants. Many of the regenerated plants showed somaclonal variation and selections were made for high active principle yielding cell lines. Protoplast fusion has been plant is regenerated, micropropragation techniques can be used to multiply and clone the desired species. Gene transfer is possible from wild and related species to desired cultivars through wide hybridization including embryo rescue systems.

Thus, to sum up, various components of the application of tissue culture technology would be:

- Micropropagation
- Conservation through cryopreservation
- Bioproduction of value added secondary metabolites
- Biotransformation of bioactive molecules
- Genetic upgradation for improvement
- Somatic hybridization
- Somaclonal variations
- Transgenic plants

The only limiting factor in commercialization of large number of medicinal plants has been the cost of cultivation. As for other annual/biennial crops per acre requirement of planting material is very large, cost of propagule is of major concern. Tissue culture can thus be adopted for species which are:

- Difficult to regenerate by conventional methods and the only way to save them from extinction is to propagate them by tissue culture;
- Species where population has decreased due to over exploitation and thus initial bulking of the stock can be taken up by tissue culture
- Species which show lot of variability in terms of the active principles with medicinal properties. Tissue culture of selected clones will help in sustainable harvest and fetching better prices both in the domestic and international market.
- Trees with medicinal properties or elites can be identified based on their potential of yielding higher amount of active principle.

Tissue culture protocols have been developed for several plants but there are many more species which are over exploited and need conservation through in vitro techniques. Also there are large number of species for which limiting factor in expanding the area under the cultivation is the scarcity of planting material.

Choosing Priorities

It is necessary to priotise the thrust areas to obtain the output of research efforts and other resources. Several factors help in determining the priorities. These include the distribution of flora, national or regional disease pattern, availability of modern health care etc. In addition we have to keep in mind the global priorities in developing new drugs so as to get a good financial return.

The disease pattern and the priorities have national characteristics but there are several diseases which are common to tropical areas and in fact to most developing countries. These include protozoal and helminthic infections like malaria, filaria, onchocerciasis etc. Many of these diseases do not exist in developed countries and large pharmaceutical houses, therefore, do not give high priority to develop new drugs for such conditions. There is a gross mismatch between the health needs of the developing countries and the interests of the pharmaceutical industry. These should, therefore, receive priority in national/regional plans. The above examples are only illustrative but we have to evolve our own list of priority for communicable diseases.

Primary health care usually requires comparatively milder medication and the acceptability of herbal medicines for such conditions is also much more. The main considerations should be adequate availability or possible cultivation on required scale, lack of toxicity and ease of formulation.

The global thrust areas for drugs from natural sources include disease conditions whose incidence is increasing and where the modern drugs are either unavailable or unsatisfactory. Some examples of such maladies may be summarised as follows:

- Tropical diseases; antimalarial, anti-filarials and anti-leishmaniasis
- Chronic conditions: anti-arthritic agents, anti-rheumatic agents
- Immunomodulators, immunostimulants, adaptogens
- Hepatoprotectors
- Rapid wounds and ulcer healing agents

- Central stimulating or sedating agents
- Alzheimers disease: prospective agents
- Memory enhancers
- Analgesics
- Sedatives

In considering the validation of the claims of ethnomedical therapies and derived preparations for introduction into the health-care systems, following deserve consideration:

(a) The inadequacy of animal models to serve as adequate systems to assess biological activities that can be extrapolated to the human situation. This is particularly so in some of the disease conditions for which no satisfactory modern therapy exists.

(b) The minimizing of toxicity tests needed to introduce the drug into a health care system. This is particularly necessary when the drug has been in long human use, toxic manifestations could be assessed by studying its long term effect on patients already undergoing treatment in the traditional milieu and the mode of industrial processing does not significantly vary from the ethnomedical methods. Product comparisons by modern instrumental parameters can also be made as between processed product and ethnomedical preparation.

(c) Clinical trials conducted under the supervision of competent authorities (*e.g.* WHO) must be a necessary prerequisite.

(d) Stimulation of traditional processing methods, as well as adherence to ethnomedical regiments will be most helpful in not missing the activitiy present in an ethnomedical preparation. This will also stimulate examination of ethnomedical theories of disease with a view to interpretation of these, if at all possible, within modern concepts. (The idea particularly refers to long standing and well documented systems such as Ayurveda, Unani and the Chinese systems).

(e) The Selection of the appropriate dosage form and mode of administration should be recently based on economic parameters as well as shelf-life potential in the situations prevailing in the developing world.

(f) There is some concrete evidence that pure compound need not necessarily be the best drugs. But on economic ground as well as on the therapeutic grounds it will serve all interests well if the most appropriate processing methodology of a plant or combination of plants is examined in this light (This would also give rise to interesting researches on the synergistic and/or detoxificant effects of other constituents in the medicinal plants or non medicinal plants that are found often added to polyprescriptions used in traditional systems).

2

Herbalism

Herbalism, also known as medicinal Botany (a neologism by Dr. K. Seshagirirao, University of Hyderabad, India), medical herbalism, herbal medicine, herbology, botanical medicine and phytotherapy, is a traditional medicinal or folk medicine practice based on the use of plants and plant extracts. The bio-informatics related to this subject could be referred to as MedBotanics (Seshagirirao).

Utilizing the healing properties of plants is an ancient practice. People in all continents have long used hundreds, if not thousands, of indigenous plants for treatment of various ailments dating back to prehistory.

There is evidence that suggests Neanderthals living 60,000 years ago in present-day Iraq used plants for medicinal purposes (found at a burial site at Shanidar Cave, Iraq, in which a Neanderthal man was uncovered in 1960. He had been buried with eight species of plants) These plants are still widely used in ethnomedicine around the world.

The first generally accepted use of plants as healing agents was depicted in the cave paintings discovered in the Lascaux caves in France, which have been radiocarbon dated to between 13,000 - 25,000 BC. Anthropologists theorize that over time, and with trial and error, a small base of knowledge would have been acquired within early tribal communities.

As this knowledge base expanded over the generations, the specialized role of the herbalist emerged. The process would likely have occurred in varying manners within a wide diversity of cultures.

Plants have an almost limitless ability to synthesize aromatic substances, most of which are phenols or their oxygen-substituted derivatives such as tannins. Most are secondary metabolites, of which at least 12,000 have been isolated, a number estimated to be less than 10% of the total. In many cases, these substances (esp. alkaloids) serve as plant defense mechanisms against predation by microorganisms, insects, and herbivores. Many of the herbs and spices used by humans to season food yield useful medicinal compounds.

The use of and search for drugs and dietary supplements derived from plants have accelerated in recent years. Pharmacologists, microbiologists, botanists, and natural-products chemists are combing the Earth for phytochemicals and leads that could be developed for treatment of various diseases. In fact, approximately 25% of modern drugs used in the United States have been derived from plants.

The use of herbs to treat disease is almost universal among non-industrialized societies. A number of traditions came to dominate the practice of herbal medicine in the Western world at the end of the twentieth century:

- The Western, based on Greek and Roman sources,
- The Ayurvedic from India, and
- Chinese herbal medicine (Chinese herbology).
- Shamanic Herbalism
- Simple Herbalism

Many of the pharmaceuticals currently available to Western physicians have a long history of use as herbal remedies, including opium, aspirin, digitalis, and quinine. The World Health Organization (WHO) estimates that 80 percent of the world population, presently use herbal medicine for some aspect of primary health care. Herbal medicine is a major component in all traditional medicine systems and a common element in Ayurvedic, homeopathic, naturopathic, traditional Chinese medicine, and Native American Indian medicine.

According to the WHO, 74% of 119 modern plant-derived pharmaceutical medicines are used in ways that correlated directly with their traditional uses. Major pharmaceutical companies are currently conducting extensive research on plant materials gathered from the rainforests and other places for possible new pharmaceuticals.?

Biological Background

All plants produce chemical compounds as part of their normal metabolic activities. These can be split into primary metabolites, such as sugars and fats, found in all plants, and secondary metabolites found in a smaller range of plants, some only in a particular genus or species.

The autologous functions of secondary metabolites are varied. For example, as toxins to deter predation, or to attract insects for pollination. It is these secondary metabolites which can have therapeutic actions in humans and which can be refined to produce drugs. The word drug itself comes from the Swedish word "druug", which means 'dried plant'. Some examples are inulin from the roots of dahlias, quinine from the cinchona, morphine and codeine from the poppy, and digoxin from the foxglove. The active ingredient in Willow bark, once prescribed by Hippocrates, is salacin, or salicylic acid alpha-hydroxybenzoic acid, $C_6H_4(OH)(COOH)$. S.A. led to the development of Aspirin, acetyl-salicylic acid, originally a trade name, patented by Bayer.

In 2004 the National Centre for Complementary and Alternative Medicine began funding clinical trials into the effectiveness of herbal medicine.

Surveys of a scientific approach to herbal medicine can be found in the books Evidence-based herbal medicine, and Herbal and traditional medicine: molecular aspects of health.

Popularity

A survey released in May 2004 by the National Centre for Complementary and Alternative Medicine focused on who used complementary and alternative medicines (CAM), what was used, and why it was used. The survey was limited to adults age 18 years and over during 2002 living in the United States. According to this survey, herbal therapy, or use of natural products other than vitamins and minerals, was the most commonly used CAM therapy (18.9%) when all use of prayer was excluded.

Herbal remedies are most common in Europe. In Germany, the term apothecary (Apotheke) is still used, and next to prescription drugs one can order essential oils, herbal extracts, or herbal teas. It is even seen as a preferred treatment over the unnecessary overuse of industrialized production of chemical medication.

In the United Kingdom, the training of medical herbalists is undertaken in private colleges. Recently, Bachelor of Science degrees in herbal medicine are offered at Universities such as University of East London, Middlesex University, University of Central Lancashire, University of Westminster, University of Lincoln and Napier University in Edinburgh.

At UCLAN the training of medical herbalists is extensive, and involves the study of anatomy, physiology, biochemistry, pathology, differential diagnosis etc. This enables the herbalist to be able to talk on equal terms with conventional medical practitioners. They learn about when they can treat, and when they should refer. They study the biochemistry of the body and the chemistry and structure of plants. Alongside this, they study traditional herbal medicine: Indications and Actions, and Energetics. They learn to recognise where conventional medical opinion diverges from traditional herbal medicine doctrine. They look at lots of different models for health care. A significant amount of self reflection is required. A medical herbalist is trained to view a situation from multiple perspectives in a non-dogmatic way.

Types of Herbal Medicines

Medicinal plants can be used by anyone, for example as part of a salad, an herbal tea or supplement, although some herbs considered dangerous are restricted from sale to the public. Sometimes such herbs are provided to professional herbalists by specialist companies. Many herbalists, both professional and amateur, often grow or wildcraft their own herbs. Many common weeds have medicinal properties (*e.g.* dandelion).

In the herbal "Healing Wise" by Susun S Weed, the three traditions of healing include" the Wise Woman Tradition, the Heroic Tradition, and the Scientific Tradition. The Scientific tradition relies on use of herbal medicines in the form of isolating the active ingredients in herbs, many modern pharmaceuticals are derived from isolating active ingredients from herbs. The Heroic Tradition relies on the belief that the body is dirty and must be cleansed, it promoted the use of purifying herbs and diuretics.

The Wise Woman Tradition uses herbs to nourish and tonify the body, herbs are used in the most natural forms possible, and they are used to support the body in healing itself. Learn more about the Wise Woman Tradition of healing with Herbal Medicine from this article, which includes the Six Steps of Healing by Susun Weed

Medicinal herbs can be used in various forms:

Herbal Teas

There are two methods of making herbal teas, infusion and decoction. Infusion is steeping lighter parts of the plant (leaves, flowers, light stems) in boiled water for four to eight hours. Decoction is boiling tougher parts, such as roots or bark for a longer period of time. Herbal teas are often used as a home remedy, and as an alternative to tea and coffee.

Some popular herbal teas include borage, chamomile, dandelion, elderflower, hibiscus, nettle, and various species of mint. Each herb has unique medicinal properties, and a range of secondary effects; and this is linked to its use as a casual drink. For instance, Borage can be used medicinally (amongst other things) as an aid against depression; and it may be drunk more casually to lift the spirits. It was traditionally served as a pep drink for weary travellers. Secondary effects include use as an anti-inflammatory or balsam; and hormonal and metabolic regulation. Other herbs may have similar side-effects, but in different proportions and are used in different ways.

Mixing Herbs: To counteract the various complications and side-effects of an ailment, or to produce a more rounded taste, a number of herbs may be mixed. A well-known mixture used against a cold includes eucalyptus leaf, mint leaf (which contains Menthol) and juniper berry. Another is the age-old favourite "dandelion and burdock", from which the popular fizzy drink was derived.

Fresh or Dried? Many flower and leaf herbs lose volatile compounds within a few hours, as the juices and oils evaporate, the scent leaks away, and the chemicals change their form. Drying concentrates other compounds as water is removed. Most herbal traditions use dried material and the reported effects for each herb tend to be based upon dried herbs unless otherwise specified.

If you are using fresh herbs, you will need more of them, and the tea will have a somewhat different effect. Finely chop the leaf immediately before using it.

Generic Western Tea is usually the leaf of one specific plant, Camelia Sinensis, which grows mainly in India and China. It can be seen as just one of many herbal teas. It is a stimulant, and its main property is to increase alertness, along with a slightly sedative or calming effect. But unlike a fresh herbal tea, it may include artificial additives to enhance the taste and to preserve it in the shops. More expensive recipes include Darjeeling (from Darjeeling in India) and Earl Grey (which has bergamot added).

Making a Nourishing Herbal Infusion

Typically, one ounce by weight (about a cup by volume) of dried herb is placed in a quart jar which is then filled to the top with boiling water, tightly lidded and allowed to steep for 4-10 hours. After straining, a cup or more is consumed, and the remainder chilled to slow spoilage. Drinking 2-4 cups a day is usual. Since the minerals and other phytochemicals in nourishing herbs are made more accessible by drying, dried herbs are considered best for infusions.

Stinging nettle (Urtica dioica) builds energy, strengthens the adrenals, and is said to restore youthful flexibility to blood vessels. A cup of nettle infusion contains 500 milligrams of calcium plus generous amounts of bone-building magnesium, potassium, silicon, boron, and zinc. It is also an excellent source of vitamins A, D, E, and K. For flexible bones, a healthy heart, thick hair, beautiful skin, and lots of energy, make friends with sister stinging nettle. It may make you feel so good you'll jump up and exercise.

Oatstraw (Avena sativa) reduces high cholesterol, increases libido, and strengthens the nerves. A cup of oatstraw infusion contains more than 300 milligrams of calcium plus generous amounts of many other minerals. Its steroidal saponins nourish the pancreas and liver, improving digestion and stabilizing moods. Oatstraw is best known however for its ability to enhance libido and mellow the mood. Do be careful whom you share it with, or you may find yourself sowing some wild oats. In Auryuvedic medicine, oatstraw is considered the finest of all longevity tonics.

Red clover (Trifolium pratense) is better in every way than its cousin soy. It contains four phytoestrogens; soy has only one (isoflavone). Red clover infusion has ten times more phytoestrogens than soy "milk," fewer calories, more calcium, and no added sugars. Red clover is the world's leading anti-cancer herb; soy isoflavone encourages the growth of breast cancer cells in the lab. Red clover improves the memory; Japanese men who ate tofu twice a week doubled their risk of Alzheimer's disease. Soy beverage can contain up to 1000 times more aluminum than milk, according to Sally Fallon, lipid researcher and fat specialist. She believes that "the highly processed soy foods of today are perpetuating. .. nutrient deficiencies... ."

Comfrey (Symphytum) leaf is free of the compounds (PAs) found in the root that can damage the liver. I have used comfrey leaf infusion regularly for decades with no liver problems, ditto for the group of people at the Henry Doubleday Research Foundation who have eaten cooked comfrey leaves as a vegetable for four generations. Comfrey is also known as "knitbone," and no better ally for the woman with thin bones can be found. And, don't forget, comfrey contains special proteins used in the formation of short-term memory cells. Its soothing mucilage adds flexibility to joints, eyes, vagina, and lungs.

Learn more about Tea and Infusions in the article series Be Your Own Herbal Expert - Tea for you, Infusion for me.

Coffee

Coffee is prepared by roasting and then grinding up the ingredients, or sometimes by decoction. It is normally stored as a powder or as granules. This is dropped directly into the hot water. Some preparations dissolve completely, while others remain partly solid, giving the drink a gritty texture.

Where the coffee remains gritty, it must be left to infuse before drinking. To avoid the gritty texture, a machine such as a coffee percolator or French press may be used.

Generic Western Coffee is the roasted seeds of either Coffea arabica or Coffea canephora. Its properties are similar to the generic tea plant Camelia Sinensis, but it has about twice as much caffeine, a richer, mellower taste, and different additives. The roasting process eliminates caffeine, and (like tea) the darker the coffee, the less caffeine it contains. When coffee is scarce, people often drink coffee substitutes.

Herbal teas include many of the coffee substitutes, and others; but they are used here for a wide range of properties, rather than merely to simulate the taste of coffee.

Herbal Tinctures

Steeping a medicinal plant in alcohol extracts the alcohol-soluble principles into a liquid form that can be stored for long periods. Different concentrations of alcohol are used to extract different constituents of the plants. For example; resins require high alcohol content and sugars usually require low alcohol content for optimal extraction.

There are many schools of thought about tincture making. In the traditional view an herb is either steeped once (single maceration) or more than once. In a double maceration the mark (or used plant material) is removed and replaced by a new batch (using the same alcohol) thus increasing the strength of the tincture. Sometimes the mark is then ashed (burnt until ash) and added back in which increase the amount of some minerals in the tincture.

In the scientific model tincture strengths are measured by a ratio of herb to alcohol (1:5 and 1:2 are the most common where the 1:2 is the stronger tincture). Many tinctures use a combination of vegetable glycerine and alcohol to extract which changes the compounds that are extracted. Herbalists often mix several herbal tinctures to form an individualized prescription for each patient.

Plant tinctures are also the basis for many homeopathic medicines. Herbal medicine and homeopathic medicine should not be confused with one another as they are very different. For a step by step instruction on how to make & use herbal tinctures visit the article series, Be Your Own Herbal Expert-How to Make Tinctures

Fluid Extracts

Fluid extracts are stronger than herbal tinctures, and can be preserved with alcohol or glycerin. They are just highly concentrated tinctures, made by distilling off some of the alcohol used in the tincture process. The final result is a liquid plant compound that can be 40 times more potent than a tincture.

Note: glycerates are herbal extracts that use glycerin as the sole extractant. They are very different and often have completely different medicinal properties than alcohol extracts. Tinctures or fluid extracts that are alcohol free should have the alcohol removed after the extraction process and replaced with glycerin which then acts just as the preservative.

Solid Extracts

Solid extracts are made from tinctures just like fluid extracts, but the entire solvent is separated from the plant compound, leaving a soft paste-like solid exract or a dry solid extract that is often as much as 400 times more potent than tinctures. Solid extracts can be diluted back to either fluid extracts or tinctures.

Many solid extracts are made in the way that apple butter is made, by simply cooking the plant material and water slowly over low heat until it forms a paste. Sometimes these are sold with a preservative added (glycerine is the most common), and sometimes they need to be refrigerated when they are opened (like apple butter).

Herbal Poultices

Poultices are a solid, vegetable fat-based mixture used externally. They have the shortest life span of any herbal remedy and must be made fresh for every use.

Poultices can be made with water or just fresh ground herb. They are applied topically often in conjunction with a heat source (hot water bottle or heating pad). They are used mostly (but not exclusively) for a localized injury (sprains, strains, scrapes, burns, bruises or cuts). They are excellent for hiking injuries (where there are usually plants and not pharmacies), but can be used for many other things.

Powdered Herbs and Tablets

Herbs that are dried and (usually) certain parts are separated out then ground to a powder fine consistency. Powdered matter can then be compressed or put in an empty capsule to form a tablet. Most tablets these days are made from some form of concentrated extract and not just plain herbal powders. This method is optimal for foul tasting herbs, highly concentrated forms and for travelling.

Powders are also used simply in their powdered form. Many Chinese medicine practitioners use powdered herbs as a base for making teas. Powdered herbs are also used topically as powders where dry skin is advantageous (some diaper rashes respond bettered to powdered herbs than ointments).

Herbal Ointments

An ointment or salve is a semi-solid preparation made to be applied to the skin. Depending on the purpose for which it is designed and its method of preparation, the texture can vary from very greasy to a thick paste.

Most ointments use vegetable oils (olive and almond are common) in conjunction with a thickener like bees wax. The herbs are often extracted in the oils for months before they are ready to be made into an ointment. The herb is then removed from the oil and it is slowly heated with bees wax to form the desired consistency. Vitamin E and essential oils are often used to preserve the salve or ointment.

The simplest ointments use petroleum jelly as a base. In traditional ointments, a combination of carrier oils is used that helps them to be absorbed through the skin, plus hardening agents to create the desired texture.

Essential Oils

Extraction of volatile liquid plant materials and other aromatic compounds from plants gives essential oils. These plant oils may be used internally in some forms of herbal medicine as well as in aromatherapy and generally for their perfume, although their medicinal use as a natural treatment (alternative medicine) has proved highly efficacious in the treatment of headache and muscle pain, joint pain and certain skin diseases.

Herbal Supplements

Herbal supplements tend to be commercial products in tablet or capsule form manufactured and marketed by the health food industry for sale in retail outlets to the general public, although there are some types that are sold only to healthcare practitioners for prescription.

Herbal supplements are often standardized to contain stated levels of active phytochemicals. Standardization can be done in a number of different ways. Many companies extract the supposedly active constituents and add them back into a base like rice fiber. This is no longer an herbal preparation as the whole herb is no longer present. Some companies follow the same procedure but add the extracted constituent to whole powdered herb. Some companies simply concentrate their whole herb until the desired constituent concentration is reached.

Many herbalists do not agree with the extraction/ standardization of active ingredients, preferring instead to use the whole plant.

Examples of Herbal Medicine

The following text needs to be harmonized with text in the article List of medicinal herbs. There are hundreds of herbal remedies. An experienced practitioner can offer a comprehensive holistic approach to health. Examples of some commonly used herbal medicines:

- Artichoke and several other plants reduced total serum cholesterol levels in preliminary studies.
- Black cohosh and other plants that contain phytoestrogens (plant molecules with estrogen activity) have some benefits for treatment of symptoms resulting from menopause.
- Echinacea extracts limit the length of colds in some clinical trials, although some studies have found it to have no effect at lower dosages than are normally given by herbalists.
- Garlic lowers total cholesterol levels, mildly reduces blood pressure, reduces platelet aggregation, and has antibacterial properties. It also has strong anti-viral and anti-fungal properties.
- Grapefruit seed extract as a natural antimicrobial has minimal effectiveness as an anti-bacterial, anti-parasitic, and anti-fungal herb.
- Nigella sativa (Black cumin) is a general medicinal plant used for diverse ailments such as cough, pulmonary infections, asthma, influenza, allergy, hypertension and stomach ache. The seeds are considered carminative, stimulant, diuretic and galactogogue. It is often taken with honey. Seed powder or oil is externally applied for eruptions of skin.
- Pawpaw used for insecticidal purposes (killing lice, worms), as well as cancer treatment and viral infections.
- Peppermint tea for problems with the digestive tract, including irritable bowel syndrome and nausea.
- Rauvolfia Serpentina, used extensively in India for sleeplessness, anxiety, and high blood pressure. The first proven allopathic medicine for high blood pressure was extracted from this herb.
- St. John's wort, has yielded positive results, proving more effective than a placebo for the treatment of mild to moderate depression in some clinical trials.
- Valerian root can be used to treat insomnia.

- Lemon juice or apple cider vinegar can be used to treat acne.
- Green tea can heal scars faster.
- Lemon grass can lower cholesterol.
- Honey can be a solution for cholesterol.

Risks and Benefits

A common misconception about herbalism and the use of "natural" products in general, is that "natural" equals safe. However many plants have chemical defence mechanisms against predators that can have adverse or lethal effects on humans. Examples are poison hemlock and nightshade, which can be deadly, although they are not sold as herbs. Herbs can also have undesirable side-effects just as pharmaceutical products can. These problems are exacerbated by lack of control over dosage and purity. Furthermore, if given in conjunction with drugs, there is danger of 'summation', where the herb and the drug have similar actions and add together to make an 'overdose'. In animals, there are other dangers. There may be residues in food from farm animals (*e.g.* eggs, milk, meat) or danger of 'doping' in competition animals. The latter may also apply to human athletes.

There is a danger that herbal remedies will be used in place of other medical treatments which have been scientifically tested for safety and efficacy, resulting in the development or worsening of a medical condition which could have been better prevented or treated. There is also a danger that an herbal remedy may itself cause harm which is unanticipated due to a lack of a full understanding of its composition and biochemical effects.

In the UK, the profession's governing bodies such as The College of Phytotherapy Practitioners and The National Institute of Medical Herbalists offer membership, education and certification. A qualified Herbalist will have studied for four years and passed exams in botanical and medical subjects. He or she will be expected to have the required knowledge to prescribe and dispense herbs tailored to the individual, taking into account their medical history and any other medication.

Effectiveness

As noted above, there have been scientific studies which show that certain plant products can cure or prevent certain diseases. The gold standard for pharmaceutical testing is repeated, large-scale, randomized, double-blind tests. Some plant products or pharmaceutical drugs derived from them are incorporated into mainstream medicine. To recoup the considerable costs of testing to the regulatory standards, the substances are patented by pharmaceutical companies and sold for high profit. Pharmaceutical firms argue that the regulations protect public safety. Cynics point out that they have a secondary effect of setting a high financial barrier to competition.

Most herbal traditions have accumulated knowledge without modern scientific controls to distinguish between the placebo effect, the body's natural ability to heal itself, and the actual benefits of the herbs themselves. Many herbs have shown positive results in in-vitro, animal model or small-scale clinical tests. The few randomized, double-blind tests that receive attention in mainstream medical publications are often questioned on methodological grounds or interpretation. Studies tend to carry more weight if they are performed in the same country as the medical scientists evaluating them. Likewise, studies published in wide circulation magazines such as JAMA receive more consideration than those published in specialized herbal journals.

Fortunately there is now much scientific research into the action and effectiveness of herbal remedies and many are justifying their traditional use. High quality trials involving proper controls and double blind methods are being increasingly carried out, with many useful results.

Herbalists tend to use parts of plants, such as the roots or leaves but not isolate particular phytochemicals. They argue that the synergy of the combined substances enhances the efficacy and dilutes toxicity. Western medicine on the other hand prefers single ingredients on the grounds that dosage can be more easily quantified. Dosage is in general an outstanding issue for herbal treatments: while most conventional medicines are heavily tested to determine the most effective and safest dosages (especially in relation to things like body weight, drug interactions, etc.), there are few established dosage standards for various herbal treatments on the market. Furthermore, herbal medicines taken in whole form cannot generally guarantee a consistent dosage or drug quality (since certain samples may contain more or less of a given active ingredient).

The issue of regulation is an area of continuing controversy in the EU and USA. On one end of the spectrum, some herbalists and consumers maintain that traditional remedies that have a long history of use do not require the level of safety testing as xenobiotics or single ingredients in an artificially concentrated form. On the other hand, others are in favour of legally enforced quality standards, safety testing and prescription by a qualified practitioner.

Some professional herbalist organizations have made statements calling for a category of regulation for herbal products. Yet others agree with the need for more quality testing but believe it can be managed through reputation without government intervention. Clearly the full debate involves issues of politics, economics and the role of government that are beyond the scope of this article.

Name Confusion

The common names of herbs (folk taxonomy) may not reflect differences in scientific taxonomy, and the same (or a very similar) common name might group together different plant species with different effects. For example, in 1993 in Belgium, in a formula created by medical doctors including some TCM herbs for weight loss, one herb (Stephania tetrandra) was swapped for another (Aristolochia fangchi) whose name in Chinese was extremely similar but which contained higher levels of a renal toxin, aristolochic acid; this quid pro quo resulted in 105 cases of kidney damage.

Note that neither herb used in a TCMcontext would be used for weight loss or given for long periods of time. In Chinese medicine these herbs are used for certain forms of acute arthritis and edema.

Standards and Quality Control

The legal status of herbal ingredients varies by country. For example, Ayurvedic herbal products may contain levels of heavy metals that are considered unsafe in the U.S., but heavy metals are considered therapeutic in Ayurvedic medicine.

In the United States, most herbal remedies are regulated as dietary supplements. Many herbs for home use could also be grown in a small home garden.

In the UK, herbal remedies that are bought over the counter are regulated as supplements,as in the US. However, herbal remedies prescribed and dispensed by a qualified Medical Herbalist, after a personal consultation, are regulated as medicines. A Medical Herbalist can prescribe some herbs which are not available over the counter, covered by Schedule III of the Medicines Act, for example. Forthcoming changes to laws regulating Herbal products in the UK, are intended to ensure the quality of herbal products used. Most Medical Herbalists will be using herbal products from a supplier who already meets these standards.

Medical Interaction

In consultation with a physician, usage of herbal remedies should be clarified, as some herbal remedies have the potential to cause adverse drug interactions when used in combination with various prescription and over-the-counter pharmaceuticals. Dangerously low blood pressure may result from the combination of an herbal remedy that lowers blood pressure together with prescription medicine that has the same effect. In particular, many herbs should be avoided during pregnancy. However, most herbal books alert the reader to necessary precautions.

Not all physicians may be familiar with the effects of different types of herbal medicine, but general practitioners should be able to refer patients to a specialist, or investigate the medical literature on their behalf. A qualified Medical Herbalist, however, will be familiar with most commonly used medical drugs and their modes of action and therefore will only prescribe herbal remedies which will not interfere with these.

3

Medicinal Plants in Alternative Medicine

Alternative medicine is defined as "any of various systems of healing or treating disease (as chiropractic, homeopathy, or faith healing) not included in the traditional medical curricula taught in the United States and Britain". Complementary medicine is defined as "any of the practices (as acupuncture) of alternative medicine accepted and utilized by mainstream medical practitioners". The term complementary and alternative medicine (CAM) is an umbrella term for both branches. CAM includes practices that incorporate spiritual, metaphysical, or religious underpinnings; non-evidence based practices, non-European medical traditions, or newly developed approaches to healing.

The list of therapies included under CAM changes gradually. If and when an unproven therapy is proven to be safe and effective, it becomes adopted into conventional health care and gradually ceases to be considered "alternative", since adoption and acceptance often take time. If a CAM therapy is proven dangerous and ineffective, it should cease to be advocated by CAM practitioners, although there are no clear instances of this happening.

Definitions

The National Centre for Complementary and Alternative Medicine defines complementary and alternative medicine as "a group of diverse medical and health care systems, practices, and products that are not presently considered to be part of conventional medicine". It also defines integrative medicine as "[combining] mainstream medical therapies and CAM therapies for which there is some high-quality scientific evidence of safety and effectiveness".

Ralph Snyderman and Andrew Weil state "integrative medicine is not synonymous with complementary and alternative medicine (CAM). It has a far larger meaning and mission in that it calls for restoration of the focus of medicine on health and healing and emphasizes the centrality of the patient-physician relationship".

In a frequently-cited review, David M. Eisenberg used the term "unconventional medicine" to signify "medical interventions not taught widely at U.S. Medical Schools or generally available at U.S. Hospitals."

Criticisms of the Term

Some scientists reject the above classification and to varying degrees reject the term "alternative medicine" itself.

The following three commentators argue for classifying treatments based on the objectively verifiable criteria of the scientific method, not based on the changing curricula of various medical schools or social sphere of usage. They advocate a classification based on evidence-based medicine, *i.e.*, scientifically proven evidence of efficacy (or lack thereof). According to them it is possible for a method to change categories (proven vs. nonproven) in either direction, based on increased knowledge of its effectiveness or lack thereof:

- Marcia Angell, former editor-in-chief of the New England Journal of Medicine, states that "...since many alternative remedies have recently found their way into the medical mainstream [there] cannot be two kinds of medicine - conventional and alternative. There is only medicine that has been adequately tested and medicine that has not, medicine that works and medicine that may or may not work. Once a treatment has been tested rigorously, it no longer matters whether it was considered alternative at the outset. If it is found to be reasonably safe and effective, it will be accepted."

- George D. Lundberg, former editor of the Journal of the American Medical Association (JAMA), and Phil B. Fontanarosa, Senior Editor of JAMA, state: "There is no alternative medicine. There is only scientifically proven, evidence-based medicine supported by solid data or unproven medicine, for which scientific evidence is lacking. Whether a therapeutic practice is 'Eastern' or 'Western,' is unconventional or mainstream, or involves mind-body techniques or molecular genetics is largely irrelevant except for historical purposes and cultural interest. As believers in science and evidence, we must focus on fundamental issues-namely, the patient, the target disease or condition, the proposed or practiced treatment, and the need for convincing data on safety and therapeutic efficacy."
- Richard Dawkins, Professor of the Public Understanding of Science at Oxford, defines alternative medicine as a "set of practices which cannot be tested, refuse to be tested, or consistently fail tests. If a healing technique is demonstrated to have curative properties in properly controlled double-blind trials, it ceases to be alternative. It simply...becomes medicine." He also states that "There is no alternative medicine. There is only medicine that works and medicine that doesn't work."

Other well-known proponents of evidence-based medicine, such as the Cochrane Collaboration and Edzard Ernst, Professor of Complementary Medicine at the University of Exeter, use the term "alternative medicine" but agree with the above commentators that all treatments, whether "mainstream" or "alternative", ought to be held to standards of the scientific method. Oxford University Press publishes a peer-reviewed journal entitled Evidence-based Complementary and Alternative Medicine (eCAM).

Regulation

Jurisdiction differs concerning which branches of alternative medicine are legal, which are regulated, and which (if any) are provided by a government-controlled health service or reimbursed by a private health medical insurance company.

A number of alternative medicine advocates disagree with the restrictions of government agencies that approve medical treatments (such as the American Food and Drug Administration) and the agencies' adherence to experimental evaluation methods. They claim that this impedes those seeking to bring useful and effective treatments and approaches to the public, and protest that their contributions and discoveries are unfairly dismissed, overlooked or suppressed. Alternative medicine providers often argue that health fraud should be dealt with appropriately when it occurs.

In India, which is the home of several alternative systems of medicines, Ayurveda, Siddha, Unani, and Homeopathy are licenced by the government, despite lack of reputable scientific evidence. Naturopathy will also be licensed soon because several Universities now offer bachelors degrees in it. Other activities connected with AM/CM, such as Panchakarma and massage therapy related to Ayurveda are also licenced by the government now.

Contemporary Use of Alternative Medicine

Edzard Ernst wrote in the Medical Journal of Australia that "about half the general population in developed countries use complementary and alternative medicine (CAM)." A survey released in May 2004 by the National Centre for Complementary and Alternative Medicine, part of the National Institutes of Health in the United States, found that in 2002, 36% of Americans used some form of alternative therapy in the past 12 months, 50% in a lifetime - a category that included yoga, meditation, herbal treatments and the Atkins diet. If prayer was counted as an alternative therapy, the figure rose to 62.1%. 25% of people who use CAM do so because medical professional suggested it. Another study suggests a similar figure of 40%. A British telephone survey by the BBC of 1209 adults in 1998 shows that around 20% of adults in Britain had used alternative medicine in the past 12 months.

The use of alternative medicine appears to be increasing, as a 1998 study showed that the use of alternative medicine had risen from 33.8% in 1990 to 42.1% in 1997. In the United

Kingdom, a 2000 report ordered by the House of Lords suggested that "...limited data seem to support the idea that CAM use in the United Kingdom is high and is increasing."

Support for Alternative Medicine

Alternative therapies provide some services not available from conventional medicine. Examples are patient empowerment, treatment methods that support the biopsychosocial model of health, palliative care and preventive health services that are not typically a part of conventional medicine,

Salient Features of Alternative Medicines

Efficacy: Advocates of alternative medicine hold that the various alternative treatment methods are effective in treating a wide range of major and minor medical conditions, and contend that recently published research (such as Michalsen, 2003, Gonsalkorale 2003, and Berga 2003) proves the effectiveness of specific alternative treatments. They assert that a PubMed search revealed over 370,000 research papers classified as alternative medicine published in Medline-recognized journals since 1966 in the National Library of Medicine database. See also Kleijnen 1991, and Linde 1997.

Advocates of alternative medicine hold that alternative medicine may provide health benefits through patient empowerment, by offering more choices to the public, including treatments that are simply not available in conventional medicine:

"Most Americans who consult alternative providers would probably jump at the chance to consult a physician who is well trained in scientifically based medicine and who is also open-minded and knowledgeable about the body's innate mechanisms of healing, the role of lifestyle factors in influencing health, and the appropriate uses of dietary supplements, herbs, and other forms of treatment, from osteopathic manipulation to Chinese and Ayurvedic medicine. In other words, they want competent help in navigating the confusing maze of therapeutic options that are available today, especially in those cases in which conventional approaches are relatively ineffective or harmful."

It must be added though that most practitioners do not hold a degree in official medicine or even have a solid understanding of scientific principles, as can be deduced from many of their publications. And providing more choice has no bearing as to the efficacy of the proposed treatment.

Although advocates of alternative medicine acknowledge that the placebo effect may play a role in the benefits that some receive from alternative therapies, they point out that this does not diminish their validity. Researchers who judge treatments using the scientific method are concerned by this viewpoint, since, according to standard controlled studies, it is an acknowledgement of the inefficacy of alternative treatments.

Danger Reduced when Used as a Complement to Conventional Medicine

A major objection to alternative medicine is that it may be done in place of conventional medical treatments. As long as alternative treatments are used alongside standard conventional medical treatments, most medical doctors find most forms of complementary medicine acceptable. Consistent with previous studies, the CDC recently reported that the majority of individuals in the United States (*i.e.*, 54.9%) used CAM in conjunction with conventional medicine.

It would be ideal for patients to inform their medical doctor when they are using alternative medicine. Some alternative treatments may interact with orthodox medical treatments, and such potential conflicts should be explored in the interest of the patient. However, many conventional practitioners are biased or uninformed about alternatives, and the exhortations to disclose alternative treatments to one's doctor do not address the complexities involved. Patients are often reluctant to share this information with their medical doctors since they fear it will hurt their patient-doctor relationship.

The issue of alternative medicine interfering with conventional medical practices is minimized when it is only turned to after the conventional medicine path has been exhausted. Many patients believe alternative medicine can help in coping with chronic illnesses for which conventional medicine offers no cure and only management. It is becoming more common for a patient's own MD to suggest alternatives when they cannot offer a treatment.

There are also the patients who have made it a habit to turn to alternatives for non-threatening disorders that may only need medical intervention in rare recalcitrant cases. They typically utilize mainstream medicine for diagnosis and basic information, while turning to alternatives for what are believed to be health-enhancing measures.

Criticism of Alternative Medicine

Due to the wide range of therapies that are considered to be "alternative medicine" few criticisms apply across the board, except possibly that of not being scientifically supported or even testable. Criticisms directed at specific branches of alternative medicine range from the fairly minor (conventional treatment is believed to be more effective in a particular area) to incompatibility with the known laws of physics (for example, in homeopathy). Critics argue that alternative medicine practitioners may not have an accredited medical degree or be licensed physicians or general practitioners and make sweeping claims without demonstrated expertise. This cannot always be considered a serious criticism, because unless a new system of medicine becomes established, it does not receive accreditation of any kind, except by its own professional organizations. This is the route homeopathy, ayurveda, siddha, unani, and naturopathy had to follow in those countries where it is now offered by accredited institutions. Proponents of the various forms of alternative medicine reject criticism as being founded in prejudice, financial self-interest, or ignorance. Refutations of criticism sometimes take the form of an appeal to nature.

Efficacy

Lack of proper testing: Evidence-based medicine (EBM) applies the scientific method to medical practice, and aims for the ideal that healthcare professionals should make "conscientious, explicit, and judicious use of current best evidence" in their everyday practice. Prof. Edzard Ernst is a notable proponent of applying EBM to CAM.

Although proponents of alternative medicine often cite the large number of studies which have been performed, critics point out the fact that there are no statistics on exactly how many of these studies were controlled, double-blind peer-reviewed experiments or how many produced results supporting alternative medicine or parts thereof.

They contend that many forms of alternative medicine are rejected by conventional medicine because the efficacy of the treatments has not been demonstrated through double-blind randomized controlled trials; this is not a moot point, since all conventional drugs reach the market only after such trials have proved their efficacy. One is led to wonder why whole categories of drugs or treatments should be excused from these routine tests. Also, some skeptics of alternative practices point out that a person may attribute symptomatic relief to an otherwise ineffective therapy due to the natural recovery from or the cyclical nature of an illness (the regression fallacy), the placebo effect, or the possibility that the person never originally had a true illness.

Problems with known tests and studies: Critics contend that observer bias and poor study design invalidate the results of many studies carried out by alternative medicine promoters.

A review of the effectiveness of certain alternative medicine techniques for cancer treatment, while finding that most of these treatments are not merely "unproven" but are proven not to work, notes that several studies have found evidence that the psychosocial treatment of patients by psychologists is linked to survival advantages (although it comments that these results are not consistently replicated). The same review, while specifically noting that "complementary therapies for cancer-related symptoms were not part of this review", cites studies indicating that several complementary therapies can provide benefits by, for example, reducing pain and improving the mood of patients.

Some argue that less research is carried out on alternative medicine because many alternative medicine techniques cannot be patented, and hence there is little financial incentive to study them. Drug research, by contrast, can be very lucrative, which has resulted in funding of trials by pharmaceutical companies. Many people, including conventional and alternative medical practitioners, contend that this funding has led to corruption of the scientific process for approval of drug usage, and that ghostwritten work has appeared in major peer-reviewed medical journals.

Increasing the funding for research of alternative medicine techniques was the purpose of the National Centre for Complementary and Alternative Medicine. NCCAM and its predecessor, the Office of Alternative Medicine, have spent more than $200 million on such research since 1991. The German Federal Institute for Drugs and Medical Devices Commission E has studied many herbal remedies for efficacy.

Safety

Critics contend that some people have been hurt or killed directly from the various practices or indirectly by failed diagnoses or the subsequent avoidance of conventional medicine which they believe is truly efficacious.

Alternative medicine critics agree with its proponents that people should be free to choose whatever method of healthcare they want, but stipulate that people must be informed as to the safety and efficacy of whatever method they choose. People who choose alternative medicine may think they are choosing a safe, effective medicine, while they may only be getting quack remedies. Grapefruit seed extract is an example of quackery when multiple studies demonstrate its universal antimicrobial effect is due to synthetic antimicrobial contamination.

Introduction to Alternative Medicine

We have made great strides in developing western medicine in the last century. Countless diseases were eliminated or controlled through advances in immunology, parasitology, and the discovery of antibiotic drugs and vitamins; the advances in surgery made possible by antiseptics and anesthesia; and the discovery of insulin and human growth hormones. From pacemakers to birth control plus, from kidney transplants to artificial hearts, America has an international reputation for making medical breakthroughs.

This, however has come at a cost. Modern medicine has raised expectations of people on the capabilities of the medicine. We have stopped taking an active part in our own healing. We trust the doctor to take care of us. Doctors, on the other hand, are very busy.

They spent more time filling up insurance forms, documenting case histories to ward of any potential malpractice suits or for meeting the "quality assurance requirements", peer reviews and other formalities that takes away the time available to practice medicine. Health care administration is reviewing the "productivity" of physicians and the only yardstick they can use to measure the performance of a doctor is how many patients he or she has seen or what is the "billable hours".

Among all these high technology shuffle, a fundamental factor that distinguished the healing profession from the time of Hypocrites has changed. Hypocrites viewed the treatment of disease as a dual process. One part was represented by systematic medicine; the other part was the full activation of the patient's own healing system. In the centuries since the great physician taught his students under the sycamore tree on the Greek island of Kos, there has been a shift away from the concept of the patient as the centre of the healing process. The physician has come increasingly to the fore as the dominant force.

The family doctor of a century ago was really a holistic doctor. He knew three generations of the family, and he knew that the mother's diabetes got worse when the teenager acted up. He saw the big picture. That's something conventional medicine has definitely lost. Family physicians, with their waiting rooms full of patients, claim that they simply do not have the time to give their full attention to patients as people, and that even if they had, many of them would be surprised, even irritated, if questioned about, say, their diet or their love life. Patients come to their doctors for tonics or tranquilizers, not for analysis.

Conventional medicine offers little for those suffering from back pain, arthritis, the effects of stress, and other chronic ailments such as cancer and AIDS. High-tech medicine is very expensive. It can also be dangerous. Its methods are potent and invasive, and it is frequently harmful. This tendency is nowhere more evident than in the amount of drug toxicity caused by modern prescribing practices. Adverse drug reactions are now so common that most patients will experience one sooner or later. The problem is that most pharmaceutical drugs are too strong.

The landscape is changing, though. Many have turning to ancient healing arts for an answer. Stone Age cave dwellers dug for medicinal plants, and the healing repertoire of the Egyptians included herbal remedies for crocodile bites. The Ayurvedic texts of ancient India are replete with magical treatments, botanical drugs, and charms designed to vanquish demons. Ayurvedic text written 5000 years ago, contain references to hardening of the arteries and recommended healing herbs to combat the problem.

The Chinese, who discovered smallpox immunization a thousand years before Europeans did, saw man as a mirror of the universe, infused with qi, vital energy that courses through channels in the body. Surgery began in prehistoric times: ancient Peruvians cut holes in the skulls of the living to provide disease with an avenue of escape.

In much of the world, Western medicine is too expensive, is unavailable, or is presented in a way that is inconsistent with traditional beliefs. There is an increasing sense that certain ancient and esoteric healing practices, long ignored by Western science, may in fact represent profound insights into the very nature of well-being.

Worldwide, only an estimated 10 percent to 30 percent of human health care is delivered by conventional, biomedically oriented practitioners. The remaining 70 percent to 90 percent ranges from self-care according to folk principles to care given in an organized health care system based on an alternative tradition or practice. The World Health Organization (WHO) estimates that 4 billion people, 80 percent of the world population, presently use herbal medicine for some aspect of primary health care.

Alternative Medicine: Definitions

What is Alternative Medicine? **: Alternative medicine is any form of practice that is outside the realm of conventional modern medicine. It covers a broad range of healing philosophies, approaches, and therapies. Most of these treatments and health care practices are not taught widely in medical schools. Examples are naturopathy, chiropractic, ayurveda, homeopathy and acupuncture. (A complete listing of alternative medical practices are given later.)**

What is Complementary Medicine?: If alternative medicine or therapy is used alone or instead of conventional medicine, it is called "alternative" medicine. If the treatment or therapy is done along with or in addition to conventional medicine, it is referred to as "Complementary Medicine" as the two practices complements each other. For example, many Chinese hospitals use acupuncture to reduce the pain during the surgery instead of anesthetics. This is complementary medicine. Later, we refer to the use of sesame oil as a complementary treatment for cancer. Dean Ornish uses life style changes to combat heart disease. These are all examples of complementary medicine.

What is Holistic Medicine?: Many of the alternative practices pay attention to the mental, emotional, and spiritual aspects of health, in addition to the physical body. Therapies like hypnosis and visualization claims to be able to change physical conditions through purely mental interventions. They believe that our bodies are remarkably resilient machines, capable, with some occasional prodding or intervention, of healing themselves. The name "holistic medicine" came from this unification of the mind and the body. Holistic practitioners treat the "whole person" as opposed to the individual organs of the body where symptoms occur. The importance of self care and preventing illness are stressed by holistic practitioners.

What is Natural Medicine?: Any therapy that relies on the body's own healing powers may be considered natural medicine. These include herbal remedies, diet and water therapies.

How Popular is Alternative Medicine?: According to a study in the Jan. 28, 1993, New England Journal of Medicine, 1 in 3 patients used alternative therapy in 1990. More than 80 percent of those who use alternative therapies used conventional medicine at the same time, but did not tell their doctors about the alternative treatments.

In 1990, Americans made an estimated 425 million visits to alternative health practitioners-more than they made to primary care physicians.

In 1992, the National Institutes of Health in Bethesda, Maryland, established the Office of Alternative Medicine, which devotes more than $3 million a year to exploring unconventional healing techniques such as meditation, massage, vitamin therapy and herbal therapy.

In 1993, Americans spent an estimated $1.5 billion on herbal remedies, including teas and supplements. While that's a lot less than the $13.3 billion spent on over-the-counter drugs, it's more than ten times the amount we spend on over-the-counter sleeping pills from grocery stores and drugstores.

As mentioned before, worldwide, only an estimated 10 percent to 30 percent of human health care is delivered by conventional, biomedically oriented practitioners. The remaining 70 percent to 90 percent ranges from self-care according to folk principles to care given in an organized health care system based on an alternative tradition or practice.

The World Health Organization (WHO) estimates that 4 billion people, 80 percent of the world population, presently use herbal medicine for some aspect of primary health care. Herbal medicine is a major component in all indigenous peoples' traditional medicine and a common element in Ayurvedic, homeopathic, naturopathic, traditional oriental, and Native American Indian medicine.

As more and more people are being attracted to alternative medicine, the willingness to consider alternative therapies is also beginning to spread to the health insurance industry. A few large carriers have started to experiment with covering alternative treatments. A pilot programme at Mutual of Omaha, for instance, covers the Dean Ornish cardiac rehabilitation programme, and Blue Cross of Washington has a policy that covers naturopathy and homeopathy.

American Western Life Insurance Company of Foster City, California covers naturopathic treatments, including Ayurveda, homeopathy, nutritional counselling, massage and physical therapy. The company maintains a full-time Wellness Line, staffed by trained naturopathic doctors who answer clients' health care questions. Premiums for the Wellness plan are about 20 percent lower than for the company's traditional plans, says Lisa WolfKlaln, an American Western vice-president who oversees the Wellness plan, "because we believe very strongly that if people do take care of themselves, if they take preventive measures, it's going to save us all a lot of money in the long run."

4

Medicinal Plants in Ayurveda

Ayurveda is India's traditional, natural system of medicine that has been practiced for more than 5,000 years. Ayurveda is a Sanskrit word that literally translated means "science of life" or "practices of longevity." Ayurveda was the system of health care conceived and developed by the seers (rishis) and natural scientists through centuries of observations, experiments, discussions, and meditations.

For several thousand years their teachings were passed on orally from teacher to student; about the fifth to sixth century BC, elaborately detailed texts were written in Sanskrit, the ancient language of India. For many years Ayurveda flourished and was used by rich and poor alike in India and Southeast Asia.

Manuscript page from Atharva-Veda, earliest Indian text (approx. 1500 BC) with much medical information, one of several Vedas (meaning "knowledge"), upon which Ayurvedic medical practice is based on. Ayurvedic manuals were written by Charaka, Sushruta, and Vagbhata that give detailed descriptions of the various practices. Charaka listed 500 hundred remedies and Sushruta over 700 vegetable medicines.

Ayurveda emphasizes prevention of disease, rejuvenation of our body systems, and extension of life span. The profound premise and promise of Ayurveda is that through certain practices, not only can we prevent heart disease and make our headaches go away, but we can also better understand ourselves and the world around us, live a long healthy life in balance and harmony, achieve our fullest potential, and express our true inner nature on a daily basis.

Ayurveda provides an integrated approach to preventing and treating illness through lifestyle interventions and natural therapies. It is based on the view that the elements, forces, and principles that comprise all of nature - and that holds it together and make it function are also seen in human beings.

In Ayurveda, the mind (or consciousness) and the body (or physical mass) not only influence each other—they are each other. Together they form the mind-body. The universal consciousness is an intelligent, aware ocean of energy that gives rise to the physical world we perceive through our five senses. Ayurvedic philosophy and practices link us to every aspect of ourselves and remind us that we are in union with every aspect of nature, each other, and the entire universe.

There can be no mental health without physical health, and vice versa. In Ayurveda, symptoms and diseases that could be categorized as mental thoughts or feelings are just as important as symptoms and diseases of the physical body. Both are due to imbalances within a person, and both are treated by restoring the natural balance mentally and physically. In Ayurveda your whole life and lifestyle must be in harmony before you can enjoy true well being. Lifestyle interventions are a major Ayurvedic preventive and therapeutic approach.

In India, Ayurvedic practitioners receive state-recognized, institutionalized training in parallel to their physician counterparts. The research base is growing concerning the physiological effects of meditative techniques and yoga postures in Indian medical literature and Western psychological literature. Published studies have documented reductions in cardiovascular disease risk factors, including blood pressure, cholesterol, and reaction to stress, in individuals who practice Ayurvedic methods.

Laboratory and clinical studies on Ayurvedic herbal preparations and other therapies have shown them to have a range of potentially beneficial effects for preventing and treating certain cancers, treating infectious disease, treating diabetes, promoting health, and treating aging. Mechanisms underlying these effects may include free-radical scavenging effects, immune system modulation, brain neurotransmitter modulation, and hormonal effects.

Basis for Ayurvedic Philosophy

Ayurveda is applicable to every living thing, as implied by its name, the science of life. Vedic sciences attribute life to more things than we normally do - the things such as air, wind, fire, the earth, planets, stars, etc. are all thought to possess conscience like living beings.

The basic premise of Ayurveda is that the entire cosmos or universe is part of one singular absolute. Everything that exists in the vast external universe (macrocosm), also appears in the internal cosmos of the human body (microcosm). The human body consisting of 50-100 million cells, when healthy, is in harmony, self-perpetuating and self-correcting just as the universe is. The ancient Ayurveda text, Charaka, says, "Man is the epitome of the universe. Within man, there is as much diversity as in the world outside. Similarly, the outside world is as diverse as human beings themselves." In other words, all human beings are a living microcosm of the universe and the universe is a living macrocosm of the human beings.

Siddha

Directorate of Indian Medicine and Homoeopathy: Siddha System is one of the ancient traditional systems of medicine in India. Siddhars the spiritual scientists of Tamil land are the founding fathers of this scientific system.

According to Siddha System the human body is the replica of the universe so are the food and drugs irrespective of their origin. Siddha system believes that all objects in the universe including human body are composed of five basic primordial elements, namely earth, water, fire, air and space. The human body is a conglomeration of three humours and seven physical components. The Food is considered to be basic building material of human body, which gets processed into humours, tissues and wastes. The equilibrium of humours, body tissues and waste products is considered as health and its disturbance or imbalance leads to disease or pathologic state.

This system also deals with the concept of immortality and salvation in this life. The exponents of this system consider that achievement of this state is possible by regulated diet, medicine and processing of mind by yogic or spiritual exercises like meditation and yoga.

Siddhars described 96 principles as the constituents of Human Being. They include Physical, Physiological, Mental and Intellectual components of a person. They are nothing but the manifestations of the " Five Basic Elements".

Disease: Disease is a condition in which there is imbalance in the "Five Elements, which alters the "Three Humours" which is also reflected in the seven physical constituents. The change disturbs the equilibrium and cause disease.

The basic concept of Siddha system of medicine is

"Food is Medicine—Medicine is Food"

Saint Thiruvalluvar says:

"Miginum Kuraiyinum Noi Seyyum Noolor Vali Mudhala Enniya Moondru"

"Wind, bile and phlegm three cause disease so Doctors deem it more or less"

Diagnosis:

"Noi Naadi Noi Mudhal Naadi Athu thanikkum Vaai Naadi Vayppa Seyal"

"Test disease, its causes and cure and apply remedy that is sure"

—Thiruvalluvar.

It is always essential to identify the cause for any disease to be accepted as a "Scientific method" The Diagnostic methodology in Siddha Treatment is unique as it is made purely on the basis of the "Clinical Acumen" of the Physician. He examines the Tongue, complexion, speech, eyes, palpation in a patient and he also examines the urine and stools. The diagnosis is then confirmed by the "Pulse Diagnosis". The above approach is collectively known as "Eight types of examinations". However, the Siddha Physician now also accepts the modern diagnostic methods for the purpose of diagonosis.

Treatment : The following line of treatment have been in practice in Siddha medicine.

- Using medicines like Choornam, Kudineer, Vadagam etc. made of herbs.
- Surgical methods like incision, excision, heat application, blood letting and leech application etc.
- Physiotherapy - Thokkanam and Varma, the Siddha way of Touch therapy, Medicated Oil application, Fomentation, herbal steam bath etc.
- Using medicines like Parpam, Chenduram, Chuxnam etc. made of minerals especially of metals.

Materia Medica: Siddhars, with their clarified and initutive intellect resulting from their yogic powers explored the nature and exploited the natural resources for the sake of humanity. They documented their findings about the characteristics of plants, metals, minerals and animal products. They documented all their findings in the form of poems for the use of posterity. Knowledge was transmitted from Guru to disciples. Their boundless knowledge on the properties of drugs, purification, processing, heat application, fixing dosage, toxicity, antidote and clinical application is astonishing the modern scientific world.

Significance: The Siddha System is capable of treating all types of chronic diseases especially arthritis, skin problems urinary tract disorders, infertility, degenerative disorders like osteo arthritis, Senile Dementia, disease of the liver, medicinally treatable Spinal disorders ,general debility ,diarrhoea and intractable allergic disorders. Aringnar Anna Govt. Hospital of Indian Medicine, Arumbakkam, being the premier institute in Tamil Nadu for Indian Medicine and Homoeopathy treats both outpatient and inpatient.

Ayurveda

Directorate of Indian Medicine and Homoeopathy: Ayurveda is an ancient system of medicine, which originated in northern India antiquity of which dates back to the period of vedas and this is said to be born from Atharva Veda. This knowledge has been gathered due to constant observation of nature for long years by men since the advent of civilization and cannot be attributed to any individual or a group of individuals by any stretch of imagination. Ayurveda is basically based on the predominance of three humours namely Vatha, Pittha and Kapha in the human body. Balanced state of these doshas denotes health and their imbalance produces disease.

Preceptors like Charaka, Susrutha have been benevolent enough to compile these invaluable treasure troves of knowledge to be passed on to posterity. The fact that Ayurveda has stood the test of time bears ample testimony to its efficacy till date.

It comprises of eight branches namely.

1. Kaya Chikitsa (General Medicine)
2. Kaumara Bhruthya (Paediatrics)
3. Bhutha Vidhya (Psychiatry)
4. Salakya (ENT and Ophthalmology and dentistry)
5. Shalya (Surgery)
6. Agada Tantra (Toxicology)
7. Rasayana (Rejuvenation Therapy)
8. Vajeekarana (Aphrodisiac therapy)

Pancha karma one of the areas of specialization, which has earned public acclaim in recent times, is also a part of the above branches. It enjoys popularity because of its being a hands on therapy and is very relaxing to the fatigued body and tired mind.

Unani

Unani system of Medicine has originated in Greece. It was further enriched and developed by Arabs and Persians. Hippocrates explained that the disease was a normal process and its symptoms were the reaction of the body to the disease. The chief function of the physician was to aid the natural forces of the body. He held that there exists in the body four humours that keep up the balance of it. He also laid emphasis on diet, drugs of plants, animal and mineral origin for curing the disease.

The Unani system of Medicine is based on the Humoural theory. Humoural pathology which presupposes the presence of four humours namely - Blood (Dam), Phlegm (Balgham), Yellow bile (Safra) and Black bile (Sauda) in the body. The temperament of persons is expressed accordingly by the words

Sanguine, Phlegmatic, Choleric and Melancholic according to the preponderance of them in the body. Everybody has got unique humoural constitution which represents the healthy state of humoural balance of the body. The Unani medicine plays a vital role when the individual experiences the humoural imbalance.

The correct diet and digestion can bring back the humoural balance. Its main emphasis is on diagnosis of a disease through Nabz (Pulse), Baul (Urine), Baraz (stool) etc. It has laid down six essential prerequisites for the prevention of disease. They are known as 'Asbab-e-sitte Zarooriya' viz. air, drinks and foods; bodily movement and repose; psychic movement and repose; sleep and wakefulness; excretion and retention.

The modes of treatment are as follows:-

(i) Ilaj bid-Tadbeer (Regimental therapy)

(ii) Ilaj bid Ghiza (Dieto Therapy)

(iii) Ilaj bid Dawa (Pharmaco Therapy)

(iv) Jarahat (Surgery)

The regimental therapy includes venesection, cupping, sweating, diuresis, bath (Hammam), massage, cauterization, purging, vomiting, exercise and leeching etc. Dieto therapy aims at treating certain ailments by administration of specific diets, whereas pharmaco therapy deals with use of naturally occuring drugs, mostly herbals though drugs of animals and mineral origin are also used.

Diagnosis and Treatment: The unani system of diagnosis of diseases and treatment restoring health, revolves round the concept of temperament or 'Mizaj'. The humours also have specific temperament. Changes in temperament are related to changes in the balance of humours. Any change in temperament brings about a change in the health of the individual. Thus imbalance of the harmony of humours and temperament along with failure of one or more parts of the body to eliminate pathogentic waste causes disease.

The Government recognized the merit of Unani system and attempts were made to develop it as a viable system of medicine for National Health care. The Unani drugs are cost effective, safe and widely accepted by the people of India. Therefore, the Tamil Nadu Government have established a Unani Medical College and Unani dispensaries.

Homoeopathy

Definition: "Homoeopathy is a system of treatment of the diseased by drugs usually prescribed in minute doses, that in a healthy person would produce symptoms like those of disease."

Origin: The Homoeopathy way of healing was devised by the Great German physician Dr. Christian Frederick Samuel Hahnemann in the late 18th Century. He came across an old idea of the efficacy of 'Cinchona bark' in treating intermittent fever due to its toxic effect on the stomach and conducted experiments upon himself in order to get the truth. He deduced from the experiment that Cinchona was used as a remedy for intermittent fever and it could produce symptoms similar to those of intermittent fever in healthy people, if taken for a specific period of time. The law of 'Similia Similibus Curentur' or 'let likes be treated by the likes' thus forms the basis of treatment under the Homoeopathic method of drug therapy employed to cure the natural suffering of person by the administration of drugs which have been experimentally proved to possess the power of producing similar artificial suffering or symptoms of diseases in healthy human being.

Basic Concepts : In Homoeopathy the main emphasis is on the remedial agents in illness and in health. It is a low cost system using only the non-toxic drugs. It has established a reputation for successful treatment of acute and chronic illness and in certain disease for which there is no or less treatment in other systems. Dr. Samuel Hanemann, who was the founder of this system enunciated the basic concepts and its principles in "Organon the Art of Healing" in the year 1810.

Due to various reasons like cost-effectiveness and non-toxic nature of its drugs, no side effects of easy in take. Homoeopathy is getting a very high recognition and acceptance from the people. Having its origin in the modern scientific age, it has the benefit of basing its theory and concept on demonstrable scientific principles and procedures.

It is based on the following cardinal principles:

1. The law of Similars
2. The law of Single Remedy
3. The law of Minimum Dose
4. Doctrine of Drug proving
5. Doctrine of dynamisation
6. Doctrine of vital force
7. Doctrine of Chronic disease

Among this, the most fundamental is the 'law of Similars'. This law states that the symptoms experienced by the sick person are reactions of the body which it mobilizes in order to counteract a morbid influence, be it a specific stress such as bacteria or viruses, or a non-specific stress such as climatic changes, environmental pollution, mental and emotional disturbances etc. Among the seven, first three are having more therapeautic importance and value.

Health and Disease in Homoeopathy: This system assumes that any disease symptoms, syndrome is the reaction of the defence mechanism of human body against the disease-causing agent. The symptoms are the means through which the body tries to regain its lost balance. According to it, the symptoms syndrome in a disease is not the disease per se but the reaction of the defense mechanism mobilized by the body in order to counteract a morbific influence existing in the body and causing the loss of balance of the healthy body. Thus the disequilibrium in the normal functioning of the organs of body implies sickness.

Diagnosis and Treatment: In Homoeopathy patients are diagnosed (their individual symptoms) but not their disease. As there is specific medicine for specific disease, unless the diseases are diagnosed, they cannot be treated, in other systems of medicine, where as in Homoeopathy, medicine are proved in healthy individuals are their symptoms are recorded. In order to treat the diseased individual their symptoms are to be matched with the patients' symptoms. Therefore, importance is given to the symptomatology than the diagnosis. By treating in this way, the natural defence mechanism (Immunity) of the individual is strengthened and recurrence of the disease is curtailed.

In deciding the treatment, the Homoeopathic practitioner follows the well-known principles of 'Similia Similibus Curentur'. In simple terms it means let the similar substance which can produce specific symptoms in a healthy individual cure those similar symptoms in a sick individual, although the symptoms have arisen from another cause *i.e.* Bacteria, virus etc., The cure is based on the assumption that the patient is extremely sensitive to that particular remedy and only to that remedy which can produce his/her symptomatology. Homoeopathy has a definite and effective treatment for some disease such as Diabetes, Arthritis, Bronchial Asthma, Epilepsy, Skin Eruption, Allergic conditions and Mental or Emotional disorders. Even, some surgical disease gets cured in Homoeopathy with out undergoing surgery.

Thus the sick person after taking treatment not only gets cured of his disease, but simultaneously regains a perfect state of health.

Advent of Homoeopathy in India

Homoeopathic system of treatment was first introduced in India in 1839 by Dr. J. M. Honigberger. During his visit to India, he cured Maharaja Ranjit Singh of Punjab. The Homoeopathic system of treatment spread successfully among all sections of the people. This system of treatment is economical and the medicines have no side effects.

Home Remedies - Siddha, Ayurveda & Unani

Siddha

Fever: For ordinary fever and intermittent fever the following decoction may be administered:-

Preparation: Take Nilavembu (Chiratta) leaves two handful add 2 glass of water boil and reduce to 50ml. and filter.

Dose: 1/2 glass 2 times or 3 times a day

If fever is accompanied with bodyache, 2 piece of Arathai (Galanga the lesser), one teaspoon of MILAGU (pepper) and 2 piece of CHUKKU (Dry Ginger) may be added for the above preparation. But the quantity of water to be increased proportionately.

If cough is present with fever, 10 Nos of Adathodai leaves (ADATHODA VASICA) may be added with the preparation.

Cough

(a) Take three leaves of Adathodai (ADATHODA VASICA) cut them into small pieces, and put the pieces into a vessel, add two teaspoon full of honey and fry the content until some pleasant smell comes. At that stage add the following coarsely powdered Athimathuram (Jamaica liquorice) 1 piece Thippli (Piper longum) 1 pinch Thalisapathri (Flucourtia calaphracta) 1/2 gm., Chitharathai (galanga the lesser) 3 piece then add 4 glasses of water and boil, reduce to 1/2 glass.

Dose: 1/2 glass two times a day.

(b) Take 2 glasses of water. Add the following drugs, Adathodai leaves (Adathoda Vasica) three numbers, Kandankathiri leaves (Solanum Xanthocarpum) five numbers. Thulasi (holy basil) leaves five numbers Thoothuvalai (Trilobatum) leaves ten numbers and 3 gms., of Athimathuram (Jamaica liquorice) after roughly powdering them boil and reduce into 1/2 glass.

Dose: 1/2 glass two times a day with honey.

(c) 10 gms., of the root of Thoothuvalai (Trilobatum), grind with Cow's milk and to be taken in the morning.

(d) Adathodai leaves juice 30 ml. (ADATHODA VASICA), Finely powdered Milagu (pepper) 6 gms., Perugayam (asafoetida) 1 gm. mixed all and take in the morning and evening.

(e) For Chronic cough, it will give relief when 2 gms., of chooranam (powder) which is made out of equal quantity of Kadukkai (Chebulic myrobolan, Ink nut) and "Thippli" (Piper longum) is administered in honey twice daily.

Ayurveda

Pyrexia (Fever).

1. Decoction of Parpataka herb (parpadakapul) 1/4 tumbler relieves pyrexia.

2. Tinospora (Seenthikodi) decoction with some black pepper powder will relieve chronic fevers -1/4 tumbler & 1/4 tea spoon respectively.
3. Sacred basil leaf (tulasi) juice and Leucus (tumbai) leaf juice along with some black pepper will cure periodic fevers—two teaspoon each and 1/4 tea spoon respectively.

Coughs

1. Take the decoction of Adhatoda roots with some honey and powder of long pepper-1/4 tumbler with 1/4 tea spoon and one teaspoon honey.
2. Ginger juice with honey is also a good remedy—1/2 teaspoon juice with one teaspoon honey.
3. Take about 1 pinch of Chebulic myrobalan (Kadukkai) powder with some honey or equal quantity of liquorice root powder (Athimadhuram). It cures cough with inflamed throat.
4. Leucus Leaf (tumbai) juice with honey is useful in whooping cough 1/2 teaspoonful with 1/2 teaspoon honey.

Diarrhoea

1. Take the pulp of Bael fruit (bilva) along with some sugar to relieve Diarrhoeas accompanied by stomach ache—1 tea spoon.
2. Mix equal volumes of yellow wood sorrel leaf (puliyarai) juice and butter milk and boil. Add 1/4 tea spoon of Ajowan (omam) powder. It cures diarrhoeas and dysentery 2 teaspoon.
3. Take powdered nut gall (masikkai) and mix with some honey 1/4 tea spoon. Three doses will cure diarrhoes and dysentery in children.
4. Take Nutmeg (Jadikkai) and tender mango leaves in equal parts by weight and make decoction. This is to be given with honey 2 teaspoon.
5. Powder of nut grass tubers (korai Kizhangu) and Aswagand tubers (amukara kizhangu) in equal quantity is given with honey—1 teaspoon.
6. Long pepper (arisitippili) ground with milk is to be given for three days to treat chronic dysentery—1/2 tea spoon.

Emesis (Vomiting)

1. Take powdered coriander (daniya) or cardamom (elakkai) with tender coconut water —1/2 tea spoon..
2. Give some quantity of coriander powder with rice washed water and sugar candy to cure morning sickness— 1 tea spoon in 1/4 tumbler

Constipation

1. Take castor (amanakku) root decoction with cow's milk and sugar in the morning in empty stomach—Each 1/4 tumbler.
2. Grind castor root with some butter into fine paste, Apply a little on the tongue of infants to relieve constipation—1pinch.

Emaciation and Weakness: Take equal 2 tea spoon powder of Aswagant roots with some milk and sugar or with gingelly oil. Regular in take will remove fatigue and weakness and it is an anabolic.

Tooth Ache

1. Use long pepper powder with some guggulu glu for brushing and cleaning the teeth.
2. Grind Fenugreek seeds (vendayam) with egg albumin into a fine paste and apply on the cheek (2 tea spoon.).
3. Gargle with ginger juice mixed with honey
4. Gargle with a decoction of drum stick root juice and Mustard 1/2 tumbler. (2 tea spoon Mustard).

Head Ache

1. Grind cleaning nut (tetrankotai) in egg albumin and apply externally.

5

Medicinal Plants and Phytomedicines

The past decade has witnessed a tremendous resurgence in the interest and use of medicinal plant products, especially in North America. Surveys of plant medicinal usage by the American public have shown an increase from just about 3% of the population in 1991 to over 37% in 1998 (Brevoort, 1998).

The North American market for sales of plant medicinals has climbed to about $3 billion/year (Glaser, 1999). Once the domain of health-food and specialty stores, phytomedicines have clearly re-emerged into the mainstream as evidenced by their availability for sale at a wide range of retail outlets, the extent of their advertisement in the popular media, and the recent entrance of several major pharmaceutical companies into the business of producing phytomedicinal products (Brevoort, 1998; Glaser, 1999). No doubt a major contributing factor to this great increase in phytomedicinal use in the United States has been the passing of federal legislation in 1994 (Dietary Supplement Health and Education Act or "DSHEA") that facilitated the production and marketing of phytomedicinal products (Brevoort, 1998).

The past decade has also witnessed intense interest in "nutraceuticals" (or "functional foods") in which phytochemical constituents can have long-term health promoting or medicinal qualities. Although the distinction between medicinal plants and nutraceuticals can sometimes be vague, a primary characteristic of the latter is that nutraceuticals have a nutritional role in the diet and the benefits to health may arise from long-term use as foods (*i.e.* chemoprevention) (Korver, 1998). In contrast, many medicinal plants exert specific medicinal actions without serving a nutritional role in the human diet and may be used in response to specific health problems over short- or long-term intervals.

For many of the medicinal plants of current interest, a primary focus of research to date has been in the areas of phytochemistry, pharmacognosy, and horticulture. In the area of phytochemistry, medicinal plants have been characterized for their possible bioactive compounds, which have been separated and subjected to detailed structural analysis. Research in the pharmacognosy of medicinal plants has also involved assays of bio-activity, identification of potential modes of action, and target sites for active phytomedicinal compounds. Horticultural research on medicinal plants has focused on developing the capacity for optimal growth in cultivation.

This has been especially pertinent as many medicinal plants are still harvested in the wild, and conditions for growth in cultivation have not been optimized. Wild harvesting of medicinal plants can be problematic in terms of biodiversity loss, potential variation in medicinal plant quality, and occasionally, improper plant identification with potential tragic consequences.

From the perspective of plant physiology, extensive opportunities exist for basic research on medicinal plants and the study of their phytomedicinal chemical production. This review presents a discussion on some fundamental aspects of phytomedicinal chemical production by plant cells with an overview of several medicinal plants that have received considerable use and attention over the past decade.

Products Involved in Plant Ecophysiology

The beneficial medicinal effects of plant materials typically result from the combinations of secondary products present in the plant. That the medicinal actions of plants are unique to particular plant species or groups is consistent with this concept as the combinations of secondary products in a particular plant are often taxonomically distinct (Wink, 1999). This is in contrast to primary products, such as carbohydrates, lipids, proteins, heme, chlorophyll, and nucleic acids, which are common to all plants and are involved in the primary metabolic processes of building and maintaining plant cells (Kaufman et al., 1999; Wink, 1999).

Although plant secondary products have historically been defined as chemicals that do not appear to have a vital biochemical role in the process of building and maintaining plant cells, recent research has shown a pivotal role of these chemicals in the ecophysiology of plants. Accordingly, secondary products have both a defensive role against herbivory, pathogen attack, and inter-plant competition and an attractant role toward beneficial organisms such as pollinators or symbionts (Kaufman et al., 1999; Wink and Schimmer, 1999). Plant secondary products also have protective actions in relation to abiotic stresses such as those associated with changes in temperature, water status, light levels, UV exposure, and mineral nutrients (Kaufman et al., 1999). Furthermore, recent work has indicated potential roles of secondary products at the cellular level as plant growth regulators, modulators of gene expression, and in signal transduction (Kaufman et al., 1999).

Although secondary products can have a variety of functions in plants, it is likely that their ecological function may have some bearing on potential medicinal effects for humans. For example, secondary products involved in plant defense through cytotoxicity toward microbial pathogens could prove useful as antimicrobial medicines in humans, if not too toxic. Likewise, secondary products involved in defense against herbivores through neurotoxin activity could have beneficial effects in humans (*i.e.* as antidepressants, sedatives, muscle relaxants, or anesthetics) through their action on the central nervous system.

To promote the ecological survival of plants, structures of secondary products have evolved to interact with molecular targets affecting the cells, tissues, and physiological functions in competing microorganisms, plants, and animals. In this respect, some plant secondary products may exert their action by resembling endogenous metabolites, ligands, hormones, signal transduction molecules, or neurotransmitters and thus have beneficial medicinal effects on humans due to similarities in their potential target sites (*e.g.* central nervous system, endocrine system, etc.) (Kaufman et al., 1999). As noted by Wink (1999), the development of structural similarity between plant secondary products and the endogenous substances of other organisms could be termed "evolutionary molecular modeling."

The Benefits of Phytomedicines

In contrast to synthetic pharmaceuticals based upon single chemicals, many phytomedicines exert their beneficial effects through the additive or synergistic action of several chemical compounds acting at single or multiple target sites associated with a physiological process. As pointed out by Tyler (1999), this synergistic or additive pharmacological effect can be beneficial by eliminating the problematic side effects associated with the predominance of a single xenobiotic compound in the body. In this respect, Kaufman et al. (1999) extensively documented how synergistic interactions underlie the effectiveness of a number of phytomedicines. This theme of multiple chemicals acting in an additive or synergistic manner likely has its origin in the functional role of secondary products in promoting plant survival. For example, in the role of secondary products as defense chemicals, a mixture of chemicals having additive or synergistic effects at multiple target sites would not only ensure effectiveness against a wide range of herbivores or pathogens but would also decrease the chances of these organisms developing resistance or adaptive responses (Kaufman et al., 1999; Wink, 1999).

A Perspective on Five Medicinal Plants

Of the vast number of medicinal plants used in Western and non-Western medical approaches, a small number have received considerable interest and use in North America over the past few years. What follows is an overview of five medicinal plants of current interest focusing on their biochemical characteristics and pharmacological actions of their plant secondary product chemicals.

Ginseng

The name "ginseng" often leads to some confusion due to its use for different plants with different phytochemical constituents. True ginsengs are plants in the genus Panax from which Asian ginseng (Panax ginseng) and American ginseng (Panax quinquefolium) have received the most interest for phytomedicinal use (Bruneton, 1995; Schulz et al., 1998; Attele et al., 1999).

These plants are low-growing perennial shade plants that generate a bulky storage root that is used medicinally. However, Eleutherococcus senticosis, a completely different plant not even in the genus Panax, is sometimes referred to as Russian or Siberian "ginseng." Roots from this shrubby tree, native to regions of Siberia and Northern China, were studied in the former Soviet Union as a substitute for Asian ginseng (Bruneton, 1995; Schulz et al., 1998).

Interest in the use of ginseng and Eleutherococcus sp. comes from their purported "adaptogen" or "tonic" activities. Such activities are thought to increase the body's capacity to tolerate external stresses, leading to increased physical or mental performance (Schulz et al., 1998).

Although an extensive literature documenting adaptogenic effects in laboratory animal systems exists, results from human clinical studies are conflicting and variable (Schulz et al., 1998; Attele et al., 1999; Huang, 1999; World Health Organization, 1999). However, there is evidence that extracts of ginseng and Eleutherococcus sp. can have an immunostimulatory effect in humans, and this may contribute to the adaptogen or tonic effects of these plants (Schulz et al., 1998; World Health Organization, 1999; Blumenthal et al., 2000).

The major secondary products present in ginseng roots are an array of triterpene saponins, collectively called ginsenosides (Dewick, 1997; Huang, 1999). The ginsenosides are glycosylated derivatives of two major aglycones, panaxadiol and panaxatriol (Bruneton, 1995; Dewick, 1997). At present, 30 ginsenosides have been identified of which the ginsenosides, Rb1, Rb2, Rc, Rd, Re, Rf, Rg1, and Rg2 are considered to be the most relevant for pharmacological activity (Bruneton, 1995; Dewick, 1997; World Health Organization, 1999). Different ginseng species have different proportions of ginsenosides in root tissue, and this may relate to reported differences in the pharmacological properties of these plant materials (Attele et al., 1999). Moreover, within a particular ginseng species, levels of particular ginsenosides can also be affected by environmental factors such as soil mineral nutrient supply (Li and Mazza, 1999). From laboratory studies, it has been suggested that the pharmacological target sites for these compounds involve the hypothalamus-pituitary-adrenal axis due to the observed effects upon serum levels of adrenocorticotropic hormone and corticosterone (Huang, 1999). However, it should also be noted that the overall effects of the ginsenosides can be quite complex due to their potential for multiple actions even within a single tissue (Attele et al., 1999).

Although extracts of Eleutherococcus sp. roots have been reported to have similar effects as the ginsenosides in animal systems, the active constituents may be quite different (Dewick, 1997). In Eleutherococcus sp., the active constituents are thought to be lignan-glycosides (eleutheroside E) or phenylpropane glycosides (eleutheroside B) (Bruneton, 1995; Dewick, 1997). However, the pharmacological action of these compounds remains unclear, and little information is available on their biosynthetic pathway (Dewick, 1997 and refs. therein).

St. John's Wort

The use of St. John's wort (Hypericum perforatum) for depression has its origins in the medical traditions of Europe well before the 1600s (Upton, 1998). In Germany, St. John's wort is currently one of the most widely used prescription medications for depression and is also extensively used in the United States as a non-prescription botanical supplement (Schulz et al., 1998; Upton, 1998). For the botanical medicine, the aerial portion of the plant is harvested and dried just after flowering, and then an alcohol/water extract is produced (Schulz et al., 1998; Upton, 1998 and refs. therein; Blumenthal et al., 2000).

Naphthodianthrones such as hypericin and pseudohypericin are predominant components in St. John's wort extracts, and most St. John's wort phytomedicines are currently standardized according to their hypericin content (Schulz et al., 1998; Upton, 1998). These chemicals are localized in dark glandular structures mainly located on the margins of St. John's wort leaves and flower petals and appear to serve in the defense against insect herbivory (Fornasiero et al., 1998). Although there is some evidence that biosynthesis of St. John's wort naphthodianthrones involves the polyketide pathway, few details are known (Dewick, 1997; Nahrstedt and Butterwick, 1997 and refs. therein).

The production of napthodianthrones in St. John's wort can be influenced by environmental factors such as light and soil mineral nutrients (Upton, 1998). There is strong evidence that hypericin and pseudohypericin contribute to the antidepressant action of St. John's wort, but it is unclear if this is associated with its activity as a monoamine oxidase inhibitor (Nahrstedt and Butterwick, 1997; Upton, 1998). Inhibition of monoamine oxidase is one mechanism by which some antidepressants operate to increase levels of neurotransmitters such as serotonin, norepinephrine, or dopamine (Schulz et al., 1998).

The prenylated phloroglucinol derivative, hyperforin, can also be a predominant component in extracts of the flowers and leaves of St. John's wort, and there is recent evidence that this phytochemical contributes to the plant's antidepressant action (Schulz et al., 1998). In human clinical studies, the hyperforin content in St. John's wort extracts correlated with the level of antidepressant action (Laakman et al., 1998).

This chemical appears to block synaptic re-uptake of serotonin, dopamine, and norepinephrine (Chatterjee et al., 1998). Blocking neurotransmitter re-uptake elevates their synaptic concentration. This represents another mechanism by which synthetic antidepressants may operate (Schulz et al., 1998). Whereas hyperforin also has antibacterial activity (Upton, 1998), it is uncertain as to whether or not this compound is effective in defense functions for the plant.

Ginkgo (Ginkgo biloba)

Ginkgo is the last living relative of a primitive family of gymnosperms (Ginkgoaceae); all other species exist only as fossils (Bruneton, 1995). Ginkgo trees are used as ornamentals worldwide due to their hardiness and appearance. Although the therapeutic use of ginkgo dates back about 2,000 years in traditional Chinese medicine, most medical applications only involved use of the seeds (Huang, 1999).

However, the phytomedicine used today is based upon acetone extraction of the fan-shaped leaves and a further purification of active constituents (Schulz et al., 1998). Clinical studies have supported the effectiveness of ginkgo in improving peripheral and cerebrovascular circulation (Dewick, 1997; Schulz et al., 1998; Huang, 1999; Blumenthal et al., 2000). A major use of ginkgo is in the management of cognitive decline associated with disturbances in brain blood circulation (*i.e.* vascular insufficiency dementia) that can occur in the elderly (Schulz et al., 1998 and refs. therein; Blumenthal et al., 2000). In addition, ginkgo extracts are useful in the treatment of tinnitus, vertigo, and for improving circulation in the legs (Schulz et al., 1998 and refs. therein). However, it should be noted that the effectiveness of ginkgo extracts in improving the cognitive performance of young healthy individuals is less certain.

The active constituents present in extracts of ginkgo leaves have been shown to be a mixture of terpene lactones and flavonoids (Bruneton, 1995; Dewick, 1997). Most commercial preparations of ginkgo are leaf extracts standardized to approximately 5% to 7% terpene lactones and 22% to 27% flavonoids (Dewick, 1997; World Health Organization, 1999; Blumenthal et al., 2000).

The prominent terpene lactones in ginkgo extracts are ginkgolides A, B, C, J, M, and bilobalide. Although the ginkgolides are considered to be diterpenes, and bilobalide is considered to be a sesquiterpene, the latter compound most likely represents a product of ginkgolide metabolism (Dewick, 1997). Studies by Cartayrade et al. (1997) have shown that although ginkgo leaves represent sites of ginkgolide (and bilobalide) accumulation, biosynthesis of these compounds takes place in the roots. Moreover, these authors demonstrated that for ginkgolides A to C, biosynthesis occurs in a sequential manner (ginkgolide A ginkgolide B ginkgolide C) through successive addition of hydroxyl groups (Cartayrade et al., 1997).

Pharmacological studies have demonstrated that the ginkgolides (especially ginkgolide B) represent potent antagonists of platelet activating factor, a bioregulatory molecule involved in blood platelet activation and inflammatory processes (Dewick, 1997; Schulz et al., 1998; Huang, 1999). The flavonoids present in ginkgo extracts exist primarily as glycosylated derivatives of kaempferol and quercetin (Bruneton, 1995; Dewick, 1997; World Health Organization, 1999; Blumenthal et al., 2000). These flavonoid glycosides have been shown to be extremely effective free-radical scavengers (Dewick, 1997; Schulz et al., 1998; Huang, 1999). It is believed that the collective action of these components leads to a reduction in damage and improved functioning of the blood vessels (Schulz et al., 1998; Huang, 1999; World Health Organization, 1999).

Kava

The use of Kava originated in the "Oceana" island communities encompassed by Polynesia, Melanesia, and Micronesia (Singh and Blumenthal, 1997). In these cultures "Kava" (also known as "Kava-Kava," "Ava," and "Awa") refers to an intoxicating beverage used in rituals and ceremonies, which is produced from the mashed rhizome and roots of the woody shrub, Piper methysticum. However, Kava is now used as the common name for P. methysticum as well as the phytomedicine produced from root/rhizome extracts. Worldwide, Kava is receiving considerable attention for its use as a treatment for anxiety, nervous tension, agitation, and/or insomnia. Clinical studies have shown an effectiveness of Kava that is comparable with sedatives such as benzodiazapines but without the development of either physical or psychological dependency (Singh and Blumenthal, 1997; Schulz et al., 1998).

From intensive chemical and pharmacological studies conducted on Kava root/rhizome extracts over the past century, several key active constituents have been identified (Bruneton, 1995; Singh and Blumenthal, 1997). The pharmacological activity of this plant appears to be associated with a family of styrylpyrones called "kavapyrones" (or "kavalactones") that have effects on several neurotransmitter systems including those involving Gln, GABA, dopamine, and serotonin (Schulz et al., 1998).

Whereas the kavapyrones shown in represent the predominant pharmacologically active components in Kava root extracts, a total of 18 have been identified at present (He et al., 1997). These remaining kavapyrones appear to be derivatives of either kawain, yangonin, or dihydromethysticin (Bruneton, 1995; He et al., 1997). Although details regarding kavapyrone biosynthesis are still lacking, evidence from other systems such as Equisetum arvense gametophytes suggest that styrylpyrones may arise from a triketide produced by successive condensation of two malonyl-coenzyme A (CoA) molecules with a phenylpropanoid CoA-ester (Schroder, 1997 and references therein).

This is similar to reactions catalyzed by chalcone synthase except that two, rather than three, successive condensations involving malonyl CoA are involved. Recent studies have shown that kavapyrone levels in Kava roots are influenced by environmental factors. In cultivated Kava plants, kavapyrone levels appear to increase with irrigation and mineral nutrient supplementation and decrease with shading (Lebot et al., 1999). Moreover, varietal differences in Kava also appear to have a role in determining the overall level of kavapyrone production (Lebot et al., 1999).

It is quite interesting that Kava plants are sterile and plantation production involves propagation from stem cuttings (Singh and Blumenthal, 1997). From genetic studies, it has been suggested that Kava likely represents a sterile relative of Piper wichmannii (native to New Guinea), which became distributed across the South Pacific islands with human migration and through somatic mutation became sterile (Lebot et al., 1999 and references therein). Kava's sterility combined with its limited growth habitat range (South Pacific Tropics), time required for growth before root harvest (approximately 8 years), and high world demand have raised concerns about potential over harvesting. Although attempts have been made to grow Kava in tissue culture for propagation and possible in vitro phytochemical production, little success has been achieved (Taylor and Taufa, 1998).

Echinacea sp.

Although there are 11 species in the genus Echinacea, this term is typically used to describe a phytomedicine produced from the aerial portion of Echinacea purpurea cv Purple Coneflower, roots of Echinacea pallida cv Pale-Purple Coneflower, roots of Echinacea angustifolia cv Narrow-Leaf Coneflower, or a combination of these materials (World Health Organization, 1999; Blumenthal et al., 2000).

These plants are herbaceous perennials native to North America, and were originally used in Native American herbal traditions for wound healing, infections, and rattlesnake bite (Bruneton, 1995). Use of this phytomedicine was subsequently introduced to Europe in the early 1900s, and current interest lies in its use for colds, flu-like infections, and upper-respiratory infections (Schulz et al., 1998; World Health Organization, 1999).

The most well-studied and effective versions of this phytomedicine involve the expressed juice of the aerial portion of E. purpurea and an alcohol extract of E. angustifolia roots (World Health Organization, 1999). A number of studies suggest that Echinacea sp.-based phytomedicines may be beneficial in reducing the symptoms and perhaps duration of upper-respiratory infections (Schulz et al., 1998 and references therein; World Health Organization, 1999).

Pharmacological studies (>350 to date) have provided strong evidence for effects of Echinacea sp extracts in modulating immune system capacity including stimulation of the phagocytic activity of human lymphocytes, stimulation of fibroblasts for new tissue production, increased respiration, and elevated mobility of leukocytes (Schulz et al., 1998; World Health Organization, 1999). Extracts of Echinacea sp. also appear to inhibit both tissue and bacterial hyaluronidase, and this action is thought to aid in localization of infection, preventing its spread to other regions of the body (World Health Organization, 1999 and refs. therein).

The immunostimulatory activity of Echinacea sp. preparations appears to result from the combined effects of a complex array of constituents: (a) a series of alkylamides as isobutylamides; (b) caffeic acid derivatives (cichoric acid, cynarin, echinacoside); (c) a series of polyalkynes (polyacetylenes); (d) a series of polyalkenes; and (e) high-Mr polysaccharides including heteroxylans (35,000 approximate Mr) and arabinorhamnogalactans (45,000 approximate Mr) (Bruneton, 1995; Schulz et al., 1998; World Health Organization, 1999). Pharmacological studies have shown effects of the alkylamides, polyalkynes, and caffeic acid derivatives in stimulating white blood cell phagocytosis (World Health Organization, 1999 and refs. therein; Blumenthal et al., 2000).

The high-Mr polysaccharide components also appear active in stimulating phagocytosis as well as promoting production of interferon (World Health Organization, 1999 and references therein). Furthermore, through their inhibitory effect on 5-lipoxygenase, the alkylamide constituents may provide anti-inflammatory activity. Although details regarding the biosynthetic pathways of these active constituents are unknown, the hydrocarbon portion of alkylamides and polyalkynes most likely represent desaturation products of long-chain fatty acids (*e.g.* oleic acid) shortened through -oxidation (for discussion of these processes, see Dewick, 1997). Chicoric acid, cynarin, and echinacoside most likely arise as conjugated products of caffeic acid generated through the shikimic acid pathway.

Although factors influencing the biosynthetic pathways of these chemicals are unknown, it has been shown that the phytomedicinal content of Echinacea sp. can be affected by environmental conditions (soil nitrogen and potassium) and the developmental state of the plant (El-Gengaihi et al., 1998).

Currently, many Echinacea sp. phytomedicines are standardized according to their echinacoside content because this caffeic acid derivative is a marker chemical unique to

Echinacea sp. However, such standardization does not consider the complex chemical interactions and possible synergistic effects necessary for the beneficial affects of this phytomedicine on humans.

Conclusions and Outlook

For the plant physiologist, work on medicinal plants opens up a wide range of research possibilities, and plant physiological studies would indeed have a major role to play in this burgeoning field. With only a few exceptions, many widely used medicinal plants have not received the extensive plant physiological characterization received by food crops or model plant systems. Although active phytochemicals may have been identified, in general, many pathways for the biosynthesis of specific medicinal compounds and the factors (biotic and abiotic) regulating their production remain unclear.

At present, a major concern with the use of phytomedicines regards the maintenance of consistent medicinal quality in botanical medicines (Matthews et al., 1999). Whereas the focus has tended to be on quality control in herbal manufacturing practices, variation in phytomedicinal content due to environmental effects upon secondary plant metabolism in the plant material could represent a significant factor. It is clear that understanding how environmental factors affect phytomedicinal production will be of great importance toward optimizing field growth conditions for maximal recovery of phytomedicinal chemicals.

In most cases, it is also unknown as to the extent to which levels of phytomedicinal chemical production by medicinal plants are determined by genetic potential versus environmental modulation. Here, the use of molecular markers (*i.e.* RFLP, random-amplified polymorphic DNA, and amplified fragment length polymorphism) in the characterization of medicinal plant populations for levels of phytomedicinal chemical production could prove useful for the analysis of traits and in selective breeding.

The use of molecular approaches and biotechnology could also have wide application and promise especially with regard to such topics as the modification of phytomedicinal chemical pathways. Production of medicinal chemicals in plants may be modified by overexpression, antisense expression, or cosupression of biosynthetic genes. Transgenic genes could also be introduced to modify existing pathways.

Mutational alterations and analysis could also be performed to dissect out basic components of metabolic pathways. The application of molecular approaches with medicinal plants would also benefit from the development of cell, tissue, and organ culture systems for in vitro growth and regeneration of medicinal plants. In addition, such tissue culture systems could also prove useful for large-scale biotechnological production of medicinal plant phytochemicals.

Overall, metabolic engineering could be useful for modifying or enhancing synthesis of valuable therapeutic agents present in medicinal plants. However, as the beneficial actions of medicinal plants can be related to combinations of phytochemicals acting collectively or synergistically, alteration of single phytochemical components could potentially affect the efficacy of a phytomedicine. In this respect, any work on modification of the phytomedicinal chemical composition of a medicinal plant through molecular methods would need to be conducted in conjunction with pharmacological studies on drug effectiveness.

Quality Control for India's Herbal Drugs

Ashwagandha (Withania somnifera) is often described as the Indian equivalent of ginseng - the Chinese medicinal plant that has captured a huge chunk of the global market. Yet the Indian herb is not a commercial success. One of the reasons for this is the lack of standards, which has led to a wide variation in the chemical composition of ashwagandha-based drugs. The discrepancy, detected during a recent study, occurs in herbal products of even reputable companies.

These drugs are portrayed as potent healers with a wide range of benefits like improving memory, cognition, stamina, vigour and resistance to diseases, as well as relieving tension and depression.

But experts feel that in view of the latest findings, a huge question mark hangs on the efficacy of these medicines.

The study was published in the February 2004 issue of Current Science, a journal brought out by the Indian Institute of Science, Bangalore. Entitled 'Phytochemical variability in commercial herbal products and preparations of Withania somnifera ', it was conducted by three institutes of the Council of Scientific and Industrial Research (CSIR) - the Central Institute of Medicinal and Aromatic Plants (cimap) and National Botanical Research Institute, both in Lucknow, and the Regional Research Laboratory in Jammu.

During the study, the amount of withaferin a - one of the withanolides of ashwagandha - was analysed in 10 products being sold in the market. Withanolides are secondary chemicals produced by the plant. The scientists assumed withaferin a to be an indicator of the presence of ashwagandha. They found that the amount of the chemical per gramme of ashwagandha varied from 100 per cent to merely 0.9 per cent. In nine of the products, the quantity was less than 50 per cent.

The research highlights these inconsistencies to underscore the importance of standardising herbal products. It also points out that the anomaly can only be corrected through stringent legislation, which doesn't exist in the country at present. Several factors like sources of raw materials, harvest and Post Harvest conditions, and processing and manufacturing techniques have to be regulated for controlling the quality of herbal products. But the Drugs and Cosmetics Act, 1940, which governs the herbal medicine industry, only lays emphasis on making drugs in clean factories and testing raw materials for genuineness.

G. S. Lavekar, director, Central Council for Research in Ayurveda and Siddha, under the Union ministry of health and family welfare, says: "Parameters such as chemical and biological markers should be set so that an acceptable range can be established for chemical constituents."

R. S. Sangwan of cimap, a member of the study team, suggests that ashwagandha should be marketed as a single plant product and not a traditional medicine where a combination of plants is used. While modern scientists are in favour of identifying active ingredients in herbal products and using them as medicines, conventional practitioners believe that such isolates cease to be traditional medicines.

The report has evoked a mixed response from the industry. Some companies are of the opinion that the laws should be strengthened. At the same time, there are others who claim their products are up to the mark. Paranjay Sharma, president of Shree Baidyanath Ayurved Bhawan Private Limited, says a manufacturer can only be penalised if standards exist. He feels quality control should be introduced in the production process at the raw material stage itself. Significantly, the good manufacturing practices that are stipulated currently do not deal with this aspect.

S. K. Mitra of Himalaya Drug Company says his company uses chemical indicators to ensure that even products in different batches conform to a uniform standard. Further, it conducts trials on humans to ensure the efficacy of the drugs. A senior representative of another manufacturer implicated in the study asserts: "The researchers did not find the withanolide because it could have been masked by other chemicals present in the product." Sharad Goel, spokesperson for Dabur, says: "We believe that the researchers should have estimated total withanolides, which is a widely accepted biological benchmark, for the purpose of comparing different products available in the market."

DNA Microarrays in Herbal Drug Research

Understanding the functions of genes is a major post-genomics challenge. Strategies like proteomics, transcriptomics, metabolomics are implemented to assign the role of genes in molecular networks. The gene expression profile of a cell determines its phenotype, function and response to the environment. The complement of genes expressed by a cell is very dynamic and responds rapidly to external stimuli. Therefore, analysis of gene expression becomes necessary for providing clues about regulatory mechanisms, biochemical pathways and broader cellular function. Conventional strategies for expression profiling such as northern blot, reverse northern blot, reverse transcriptase-polymerase chain reaction (RT-PCR), nuclease protection, enzyme-linked immunosorbent assay (ELISA), western blot, in situ hybridization and immunohistochemistry are optimized for single gene analysis. Although, it is possible to modify at least some of these techniques for multiplexing, the procedure becomes increasingly technically cumbersome.

For genome wide expression analysis it is necessary to develop technologies having high degree of automation, since in any living organism thousands of genes and their products function in a complicated and orchestrated way. DNA microarrays were developed in response to the need for a high-throughput, efficient and comprehensive strategy that can simultaneously measure all the genes, or a large defined subset, encoded by a genome. Several different methodologies including differential display PCR, northern blots, quantitative PCR, serial analysis of gene expression (SAGE) and TIGR Orthologous Gene Alignments (TOGA) are used alongside microarrays as research tools.

With an initial focus in the post-genomic era on tracking gene expression changes for target identification, microarray applications soon widened to span the entire drug discovery pipeline. DNA microarrays are being used to study the transcriptional profile in various physiological and pathological conditions, leading to the mining of novel genes and molecular markers for diagnosis, prediction or prognosis of those specific states.

Success in the DNA microarray field has led to protein array development. Protein microarrays are mainly applied to protein function studies, screening the production of antibodies and recombinant proteins, discovery of proteins implicated in disease or those that are potential drug targets, rapid detection or diagnosis of disease screening for protein-protein, DNA-protein and enzyme-substrate interactions. High-density human protein arrays are undermined by the incomplete knowledge of full-length human gene clones and the vast idiosyncrasies of proteins with respect to stability and structure. Although protein microarrays may not have reached the stage of maturity of DNA microarrays, recent developments have shown that many of the barriers holding back the technology can be overcome.

Recently cell-based arrays employing matrices of living cells engineered to express select proteins have rapidly emerged as versatile tools for the high-throughput analysis of gene function. Such arrays can facilitate genome-scale studies on different aspects of protein function, including biochemical activities, gene disruption phenotypes and protein-protein interactions.

Another version of living arrays called transfection microarray has been demonstrated as an alternative to protein microarrays for the identification of drug targets, and as an expression cloning system for the discovery of gene products that alter cellular physiology. A siRNA transfected cell microarray has been developed to facilitate large-scale, high-throughput functional genomics studies using RNAi.

Chemical microarrays, which are arrays of small organic compounds, represent a novel approach towards analysis of chemical libraries. They are widely used to analyze the interaction of proteins with organic compounds in a miniaturized and high-throughput fashion. Several modified technologies spanning wide range of macromolecular microarrays to cell arrays have opened new horizons in molecular and physiological systems.

The DNA Microarray

DNA microarray is an orderly arrangement of thousands of oligonucleotides or identified sequenced genes printed on an impermeable solid support, usually glass, silicon chips or nylon membrane. A number of terms such as DNA arrays, gene chips and biochips are often used to describe these devices. The DNA microarray field is a combination of several technologies, including automated DNA sequencing, DNA amplification by PCR, oligonucleotide synthesis, nucleic acid labeling chemistries and bio-informatics. Two most common types of DNA microarrays include one in which the DNA (in the form of a single stranded short oligonucleotide) is synthesized in situ using photolithographic or other techniques and another where the DNA (usually in the form of a cDNA or full-length ORF) is post-synthetically attached to a solid support.

Depending on the kind of probe (immobilized DNA) used to generate the array and, ultimately, the information that is derived from it, DNA microarrays are used for different applications. As a definition in the context of microarrays, a 'probe' is the (partial) genomic sequence of a gene deposited and fixed on the Microarray, whereas the 'target' is the biological sample material.

Although there are many protocols and types of microarray experiments, the basic steps involved in any microarray experiment are isolating RNA or mRNA from appropriate biological samples; applying a fluorescent tag to the RNA or cDNA copy of it; hybridizing the labelled RNA or cDNA (target) to a microarray (probe) for a period of time after which the excess is washed off; scanning the microarray under laser light and data analysis using appropriate software.

Natural product research is often based on ethnobotanical information and many of the drugs used today were employed in indigenous societies. One of the aims of ethnopharmaceutical research is better understanding of the pharmacological effects of different medicinal plants traditionally used in healthcare. Plants are regarded as a promising source of novel therapeutic agents due to their higher structural diversity as compared to standard synthetic chemistry. Plants have applications in the development of therapeutic agents: as a source of bioactive compounds for possible use as drugs. There are three approaches to natural product-based drug discovery: screening of crude extracts; screening of pre-fractionated extracts; screening of pure compounds.

In the past decade there has been a paradigm shift from single-target drugs to multi-target drugs. Multi-target approaches are directed toward activation of defence, protective and repair mechanisms of the body rather than destruction of the damage-causing agent. This may be achieved by the use of a combination of drugs as in AIDS, cancer, atherosclerosis or use of single compounds that affect many targets simultaneously, *e.g.* Gleevec™, salicylate, metformin, Pemetrexed (Alimta) and a multi-targeted antifolate. The concept of multi-targeted therapy exists in traditional medical treatments that employ multi-component extracts of natural products.

With the exception of pure substances, botanical derivatives obtained from medicinal plants usually contain several classes of compounds, which simultaneously act on multiple targets. However, very few herbal medicinal products have documentation comparable to synthetic drugs. Preparation of highly standardized herbal products with respect to chemical composition and biological activity is complicated due to the myriad range of chemicals. This also makes it difficult to precisely predict the molecular targets, mechanism of action and side effects of such products.

Use of validated analytical methods to quantify specific chemical markers remains the key point to obtain chemically standardized extracts. However many minor components with potential biological effects remain neglected from quantitative analysis of chemical markers. In the past years the development of assays on the level of molecules (receptor binding and enzyme inhibition) opened complete new perspectives for plant-based products as source of new drugs.

Advances in high-throughput experimentation have resulted in massive databases of genomic, proteomic and chemical data which in combination with efficient separation methods and powerful spectrometric methods for identification and structure elucidation can be used for identification of active compounds. In addition, the past two decades has witnessed a number of citations that describe a diverse range of molecular mechanisms that govern cellular behaviour. A systems biology approach that integrates such large and diverse sources of information together will serve to make useful biological predictions about the pharmacological effects of natural products.

DNA microarrays may provide a suitable high-throughput platform for research and development of drugs from natural products. In natural products a broad repertoire of chemical entities act together on multiple targets that makes it necessary to study the changes in expression of multiple genes simultaneously. Novel technologies such as SAGE and DNA microarrays allow rapid and detailed analysis of thousands of transcripts, providing a revolutionary approach to the investigation of gene expression.

In this review, we discuss the applications of DNA microarray technology in herbal drug research and development with suitable examples.

There are three main applications of DNA microarrays: first, in pharmacodynamics for discovery of new diagnostic and prognostic indicators and bio-markers of therapeutic response; elucidation of molecular mechanism of action of a herb, its formulations or its phytochemical components and identification and validation of new molecular targets for herbal drug development. Second, in pharmacogenomics for prediction of potential side-effects of the herbal drug during preclinical activity and safety studies; identification of genes involved in conferring drug sensitivity or resistance and prediction of patients most likely to benefit from the drug and use in general pharmacogenomic studies. Third, in pharmacognosy for correct botanical identification and authentication of crude plant materials as part of standardization and quality control. These applications are described here with some examples.

Herbal products are usually whole herbs, their formulations or extracts consisting of several bioactive compounds. With the increased demand for scientifically validated and standardized herbal product there is a need for better understanding of the molecular mechanisms underlying their biological activity. Although, the physiological actions of many herbal drugs are being studied at the molecular level, it remains unclear what are the targets of individual phytochemical components of herbs and how these molecules contribute to biological activities. Examples of the applications of microarray-based gene expression studies in elucidating molecular mechanism of action of pure compounds, different phytochemical groups and herbal extracts are discussed here.

The molecular pathways underlying diverse biological activity of the triterpenoid compounds isolated from the tropical medicinal plant Centella asiatica when studied with gene microarrays showed that Centella triterpenes evoke a gene-expression response consistent with their prevailing medical uses in the treatment of connective tissue disorders such as wound healing and microangiopathy.

The identification of genes modulated by these compounds provides the basis for a molecular understanding of Centella's bioactivity, and opportunities for the quantitative correlation of this activity with clinical effectiveness at a molecular level. Similarly, the antiproliferative activity of Coptidis rhizoma, a medicinal herb, and its major component berberine was investigated in human pancreatic cancer cell lines.

Gene expression patterns associated with sensitivities to each agent were analyzed with oligonucleotide arrays that comprised approximately 11,000 genes. It was possible to identify common and distinct genes related to anti-proliferative activities of purified berberine and C. rhizoma.

Involvement of genes in apoptosis inducing activity of alkaloids from Chinese medicinal herb Tripterygium hypoglaucum (levl.) Hutch (Celastraceae) root was examined using cDNA microarrays containing 3000 human genes derived from a leukocyte cDNA library. Induction of apoptosis by Tripterygium hypoglaucum alkaloids was found to be through c-myc and NF-kappa B signaling pathways.

Gene expression pattern of inferior colliculus from DBA/2J mice with audiogenic seizure and those treated with Qingyangshenylycosides, a traditional Chinese medicine, were examined. Gene expression analysis using Agilent oligo microarray showed that total of 134 genes were either up- or down-regulated during audiogenic seizure. Qingyang-shenylycosides prevented many of the audiogenic seizure induced gene expression changes.

Nevertheless, some of the audiogenic seizure induced genes were further enhanced or reversed by Qingyangshenylycosides treatment. The data provided important information regarding the molecular mechanisms of audiogenic seizure and the mechanism of action of Qingyangshenylycosides.

Oligonucleotide microarrays consisting of 87 probes representing 87 human cardiovascular disease-related genes were used to investigate the molecular mechanisms of saponins from the rhizome of Anemarrhena asphodeloides Bunge. Gene expression patterns in saponin treated and untreated human umbilical vein endothelial cells were analyzed. The results suggest that saponins may have beneficial effect on cardiovascular diseases by modulating the function of vein endothelial cells.

A gene chip, (Rat Genome U34A) was used to elucidate the gene regulatory pattern of Epimedium flavonoids in immune homeostasis remodeling in the aged rats. Expression pattern characterized by up-regulation of apoptosis promoting gene expression and down-regulation of apoptosis inhibiting genes expression, is the important gene background of immuno-homeostasis imbalance in aged. Epimedium flavonoids reverse these abnormal changes to reconstruct a beneficial equilibrium of gene expression and thus to further remodel the immuno-homeostasis in the aged.

Mechanism of herbal glycoside recipes retrieving deficient ability of spatial learning memory in mice suffering from cerebral ischemia/repurfusion was studied using DNA micoarray system. Gene expression pattern was analyzed in the groups that showed increased ability of spatial learning. A 1.8-fold increase in expression was observed for many genes (38-46) including genes in cell cycle regulation, signal transduction, nerve system transcription factors, DNA-binding protein, etc. Nine genes related to retrieving deficient ability of spatial learning memory when treated with glycoside recipes were found in this study.

Chronic cocaine use is known to elicit changes in the pattern of gene expression within the brain. The hippocampus plays a critical role in learning and memory and may also play a role in mediating behaviours associated with cocaine abuse. To profile the gene expression response of the hippocampus to chronic cocaine treatment, cDNA hybridization arrays were used to illuminate cocaine-regulated genes in rats treated non-contingently with a binge model of cocaine. Similarly, using DNA microarray analysis gene expression changes with chronic morphine and antagonist-precipitated withdrawal in two brain regions involved in behavioural effects of morphine in both mice and rats, were characterized

Si-Jun-Zi decoction (SJZD), a traditional Chinese herbal prescription, has been used clinically for treating patients with disorders of the digestive system. Previous studies indicated that the polysaccharides of SJZD are the active components contributing towards its pharmacological effects in improving gastro-intestinal function and immunity. SJZD polysaccharide was found to have protective effect and enhanced re-epithelialization on wounded IEC-6 cells.

To elucidate the modulatory effect of polysaccharides of SJZD on wounded IEC-6 cells at the molecular level, an oligonucleotide microarray was employed to study differential gene expression of treated IEC-6 cells and the candidate genes were validated by RT-PCR. There was increased expression of genes coding for ion channels and transporters, which are critical to cell migration and restoration of wounded intestinal cells, suggesting a possible mechanism for re-epithelialization.

Clinical trials on antimicrotubule agents, docetaxel and estramustine combination treatment have suggested improved antitumor activity in hormone-refractory prostate cancer. However, the molecular mechanisms involved in the combination treatment with docetaxel and estramustine have not been fully elucidated. In order to establish such molecular mechanisms in both hormone insensitive and sensitive prostate cancer cells, gene expression profiles of docetaxel- and estramustine-treated prostate cancer cells were obtained by using Affymetrix Human Genome U133A Array. Clustering analysis based on biological function showed that docetaxel and estramustine combination treatment down-regulated some genes that are known to regulate cell proliferation, transcription, translation, and oncogenesis.

In contrast, docetaxel and estramustine combination treatment up-regulated some genes related to induction of apoptosis, cell cycle arrest, and tumor suppression. Docetaxel and estramustine also showed differential effects on gene expression between mono- and combination treatment.

Combination treatment with docetaxel and estramustine caused alternations of a large number of genes, many of which may contribute to the molecular mechanisms by which docetaxel and estramustine inhibit the growth of prostate cancer cells. These results provide novel molecular targets of docetaxel and estramustine combination treatment in prostate cancer cells.

Extracts

High-density oligonucleotide microarrays have been used for pioneer studies on the multiple gene expression effects exhibited by Ginkgo biloba leaf extract EGb 761, changing traditional pharmacology and medicine concepts. EGb 761 has been known to have neuroprotective effects ranging from molecular and cellular, to animal and human studies, however, the mechanisms remain unclear. DNA microarray based analyses has largely helped in identifying its targets and mechanism of action. High-density oligonucleotide microarrays were used to define the transcriptional effects in the cortex and hippocampus of mice whose diets were supplemented with the herbal extract.

This study reveals that diets supplemented with Ginkgo biloba extract have notable neuromodulatory effects in vivo and illustrates the utility of genome-wide expression monitoring to investigate the biological actions of complex extracts. Further, DNA microarray analyses revealed that transcription of multiple apoptosis-related genes is either up- or down-regulated in cells treated with EGb 761. These results suggest that inhibition of apoptotic machinery may, at least in part, mediate multiple neuroprotective effects of EGb 761. Mechanism of cytostatic action of EGb 761 was elucidated with the help of DNA microarray and the genes important for tumour growth were identified.

Ginkgo extract and one of its terpenoid constituents, ginkgolide B, inhibited the proliferation of a highly aggressive human breast cancer cell line and xenografts of this cell line in nude mice. cDNA microarray analyses have shown that exposure of human breast cancer cells to a Ginkgo extract altered the expression of genes that are involved in the regulation of cell proliferation, cell differentiation or apoptosis, and that exposure of human bladder cancer cells to a Ginkgo extract produced an adaptive transcriptional response that augments antioxidant status and inhibits DNA damage.

A human genome screen for TNF?-inducible genes was used to identify the genetic basis of the anti-inflammatory effects of standardized Boswellia serrata extract, 5-Loxin in microvascular endothelial cells. Acutely, TNF?-induced 522 genes; of which 113 genes were clearly sensitive to 5-Loxin treatment. Such genes directly related to inflammation, cell adhesion, and proteolysis. The robust 5-Loxin -sensitive candidate genes were then subjected to further processing which led to the recognition of the primary 5-Loxin -sensitive TNF?-inducible pathways. One mechanism by which TNF?, causes inflammation is by potently inducing the expression of adhesion molecule VCAM-1. 5-Loxin was found to completely inhibit VCAM-1 expression.

Water-extract of Paeoniae Radix has inhibitory effect on the growth of both HepG2 and Hep3B cell lines. Using cDNA microarray technology and RT-PCR analysis the drug targets of Paeoniae Radix in inhibition of tumour cells growth were elucidated.

Several studies have indicated that extracts of S. barbata have growth inhibitory effects on a number of human cancers. However, the mechanism underlying the antitumor activity was unclear. cDNA microarray analysis showed that 16 genes, involved in DNA damage, cell cycle control, nucleic acid binding and protein phosphorylation, underwent more than 5-fold change. These data indicated that these processes are involved in S. barbata-mediated killing of cancer cells.

The effect of Syzygium aromaticum (L.) Merrill and Perry (clove) extract on tissues that regulate glucose metabolism was studied by analysis of gene expression using DNA microarray. The data showed that the extract acts like insulin in hepatocytes and hepatoma cells by reducing phosphoenolpyruvate carboxykinase and glucose 6-phosphatase gene expression. Much like insulin, clove-mediated repression was reversed by PI3K inhibitors and N-acetylcysteine. Moreover, clove and insulin were found to regulate the expression of many of the same genes in a similar manner. These results indicate a potential role for compounds derived from clove as insulin-mimetic agents.

A cDNA microarray study demonstrated significant inhibition of inducible endothelial CD36 expression, a novel cardioregulatory gene, by IH636 grape seed proanthocyanidin extract.

Both the prototypic tricyclic antidepressant imipramine (IMI) and the extract of St John's wort (SJW) can be effective in the treatment of major depressive disorder. Affymetrix chips were used to study hypothalamic gene expression in rats treated with SJW or IMI to test the hypothesis that chronic antidepressant treatment by various classes of drugs results in shared patterns of gene expression that may underlie their therapeutic effects. SJW treatment differentially regulated 66 genes and expression sequence tags (ESTs) and IMI treatment differentially regulated 74 genes and ESTs. Six common transcripts in response to both treatments were found. Both treatments also affected different genes that are part of the same cell function processes, such as glycolytic pathways and synaptic function. The data support the hypothesis that chronic antidepressant treatment by drugs of various classes may result in a common, final pathway of changes in gene expression in a discrete brain region.

Recently, a rapid throughput screening system involving gene expression analysis was developed in order to investigate the potential of bioactive chemicals contained in natural health products as effective drug therapy, in particular the ability of these chemicals to alleviate the inflammatory response in human airway epithelial cells. The pharmacogenomic activities of Anoectochilus formosanus extract as a crude phytocompound mixture were compared to those conferred by the single-compound drug, plumbagin in MCF-7 cancer cells. This study offers evidence to support the search for fractionated medicinal herb extracts or phytocompound mixtures, in addition to single-compound drugs, as defined therapeutic agents. DNA microarray can be used for activity-guided fractionation of herbal extracts in order to determine active principles.

DNA Microarrays in Pharmacogenomics

Pharmacogenomics is the study of genes and the gene products (proteins) essential for pharmacological or toxicological responses to pharmaceutical agents. Oligonucleotide-based DNA chip technology or cDNA microarray can be used to analyze gene expression profiles that are induced or repressed by xenobiotics.

An attempt has been made to develop microarray genotyping system for multiplex analysis of a panel of single nucleotide polymorphisms (SNPs) in genes encoding proteins involved in blood pressure regulation, and to apply this system in a pilot study demonstrating its feasibility in the pharmacogenetics of anti-hypertensive drug response. DNA microarray techniques might prove to be a reliable basis for predicting response (or lack of response) of individuals to herbal drugs.

Technologies designed to characterize genes and their products on a discovery scale are now having an impact on many areas of biology, including toxicology. Toxicogenomics is the sub-discipline that merges genomics with toxicology. In toxicology research, gene expression profiling facilitates mechanism-based research on toxicant action by comparing results for an experimental compound with a database. Recently several studies have demonstrated the utility of microarray analysis for studying genome-wide effects of xenobiotics and the rapid identification of toxic hazards for novel drug candidates.

An example of such a platform is ToxBlot II, a custom microarray containing cDNAs representing 12564 human genes chosen on the basis of their potential relevance to a broad range of toxicities. ToxBlot II allows the simultaneous expression profiling of genes representing entire cellular pathways, facilitating a very detailed investigation of potential mechanisms of toxicity. cDNA microarray analysis was used to study the expression level of genes in oral fibroblast cell lines in response to exposure to ripe areca nut extract.

The results showed up-regulation of IL-6 expression and down-regulation of PDGFR, APP-1 and KGF-1 expressions in multiple cell lines assayed. The down-regulation of KGF-1 expression in oral fibroblast cell lines potentially impairs the proliferation of overlying keratinocytes, which could partially explain the frequent epithelial atrophy observed in chronic areca chewers in vivo.

This study established a novel toxicogenomic database for areca nut extract. cDNA microarray analysis was also used to analyze the mRNA expression patterns of 1177 genes in ten oral cancer patients with betel quid chewing history. This study provides pilot data for understanding the pathogenesis of oral cancer in countries like Taiwan where betel quid chewing is prevalent.

Recent studies have highlighted that concurrent use of herbs may mimic, magnify, or oppose the effect of drugs. DNA microarray can be used for studying herb-drug interactions, and the mechanisms underlying these interactions.

Several botanical constituents in PC-SPES, a botanical preparation, inhibit tumour growth through cell cycle arrest and apoptosis. LNCaP prostate carcinoma cells were treated with PC-SPES, and changes in gene expression were determined by complementary DNA (cDNA) microarray hybridization and northern blot analyses. mRNA levels of? -tubulin decreased sevenfold. The results show that PC-SPES may interfere with microtubule polymerization.

This activity has implications for the clinical management of patients with advanced prostate cancer who may be taking PC-SPES concurrently with microtubule-modulating chemotherapeutic agents, such as paclitaxel. cDNA microarray analysis was used to identify gene expression changes in LNCaP prostate carcinoma cells exposed to PC-SPES and estrogenic agents including diethylstilbestrol. Transcripts encoding cell cycle-regulatory proteins,? - and? -tubulins, and the androgen receptor were down-regulated by PC-SPES. A comparison of gene expression profiles resulting from these treatments indicates that PC-SPES exhibits activities distinct from those attributable to diethylstilbestrol and suggests that alterations in specific genes involved in modulating the cell cycle, cell structure, and androgen response may be responsible for PC-SPES-mediated cytotoxicity.

DNA Microarray in Pharmacognosy

Use of authentic herbal materials is the first step to ensure quality, safety and efficacy of herbal medicines. DNA polymorphism-based assays have been developed for the identification of herbal medicines. In this approach, small amounts of DNA are amplified by the polymerase chain reaction and the reaction products are analyzed by gel electrophoresis, sequencing, or hybridization with species-specific probes. Recently, microarrays have been applied for the DNA sequence-based identification of medicinal plants.

To utilize DNA microarrays for identification and authentication of herbal material, it is necessary to identify a distinct DNA sequence that is unique to each species of medicinal plant. The DNA sequence information is then used to synthesize a corresponding probe on a silicon-based gene chip. These probes are capable of detecting complementary target DNA sequences if present in the test sample being analyzed.

Oligonucleotide probes specific for polymorphisms in the D2 and D3 regions of 26S rDNA gene of several Fritillaria species were designed and printed on the poly-lysine coated slides to prepare a DNA chip. Differentiation of the various Fritillaria species was accomplished based on hybridization of fluorescent labelled PCR products with the DNA chip. The results demonstrated the reliability of using DNA chips to identify different species of Fritillaria, and that the DNA chip technology can provide a rapid, high throughput tool for genotyping and plant species authentication.

Similarly, using fluorescence-labelled ITS2 sequences as probes, distinctive signals were obtained for the five medicinal Dendrobium species listed in the Chinese Pharmacopoeia. The established microarray was able to detect the presence of D. nobile in a Chinese medicinal formulation containing nine herbal components.

A silicon-based DNA microarray using species-specific oligonucleotide probes is designed and fabricated to identify multiple toxic traditional Chinese medicinal plant species by parallel genotyping. Chip-based authentication of medicinal plants may be useful as economical, precise tool for quality control and safety monitoring of herbal pharmaceuticals and neutraceuticals.

Identification of herbal materials, which commonly consist of dried or processed parts, is difficult. This is particularly true for similar looking herbal materials that can often vary greatly in their medicinal properties and market value. DNA microarray based technology can provide an efficient, accurate and cheaper means of testing the authenticity of hundreds of samples simultaneously while conventional chemical methodologies usually take several days for verification.

Chip-based authentication of medicinal plants can be useful as a tool for quality control and safety monitoring of herbal pharmaceuticals and neutraceuticals and will significantly add to the medical potential and commercial profitability of herbal products.

This application of DNA microarrays will not only benefit the herbal drug industry but can also facilitate the identification of herbal products by regulatory authorities. An international initiative, the Consortium for the Barcode of Life (CBOL) is devoted to developing DNA barcoding as a tool for correct taxonomic identification of species, including medicinal plants. DNA microarrays can provide a suitable technology platform for such an initiative.

Perspective

Traditionally, the pharmaceutical industry has focused on modifying one gene or protein at a time as the basis for identifying new drugs. The quest for a molecule to modify a single key factor in a disease process may not provide a solution for many complex diseases where multiple cell types and/or multiple pathways contribute to disease. Herbal extracts or mixtures represent combinatorial chemistry of nature with vast repertoire of chemical entities that have a complex effect on numerous cellular components and functions.

They have great potential in the multi-target approach to diseases. However, potential of herbal drugs as defined therapeutic agents is undermined by the difficulty in standardization, pharmacodynamics and pharmacokinetics of these multi-component mixtures. Microarray analysis of gene expression can be useful for elucidating the molecular mechanisms and networks underlying the complex pharmacological function of herbal extracts and mixtures. Studying the patterns of gene expression at many stages during the treatment process can reveal mechanism from a modern genetic perspective and will help to identify bio-markers of adverse or favourable response. A positive correlation between the transcriptional response induced by an herbal drug and a database profile of an existing therapeutic agent can provide insight into target specificity, mechanism of action, as well as facilitate analysis of pathways downstream of the target.

It will also help in identification of novel therapeutic applications of a herbal drug. DNA microarrays can also be used for activity-guided fractionation of herbal extracts thereby helping in narrowing down upon the active principle producing the desired effect. Microarrays have applications in the entire drug discovery pipeline to improve selection of biological targets and lead compounds. Correlation of gene expression data of herbal drug candidates with clinical outcome or bio-markers of response in biological system will facilitate selection of best candidate for drug development.

In the area of pharmacogenomics, DNA microarrays will facilitate development of individually optimized drugs based on differential gene expression patterns. Genetic polymorphism studies can be done to classify individuals according to their drug metabolizing capacities or response to disease. SNP screening of patients undergoing treatment with a particular herbal drug and correlating these data with recovery profile would help to understand which individuals or groups are likely to be benefited by the drug.

Microarray analysis of gene expression has become a suitable approach for the biological effects of drugs and other chemicals. Gene expression profile screens focused on genes that are relevant to toxicity can be useful for prediction of potential herbal drug side effects during pre-clinical development and toxicology studies. They can also be applied for studying herb-drug interactions and their underlying mechanisms.

Medicinal plants are an integral part of TM/CAM such as Ayurvedic, Chinese, Native American and many other traditional systems of medicine. Clinical experiences, observations or documented data becomes a starting point for traditional knowledge based drug development. Although the clinical existence of traditional medicine spans several generations, it may be hazardous to extrapolate from such uses to current practice, since herbs and or their formulations used may be very different from the commercial herbal products available today.

Many questions remain concerning quality, efficacy, safety, bioavailability and mechanisms of action of even the most widely used herbs. These questions can be answered by rigorous application of scientific principles in high quality basic and clinical research. There is a need for scientific validation of safety, efficacy, therapeutic claims, bioavailability and mechanism of action of these medicines that are being used in the population since centuries. Microarray based approach can facilitate high throughput, fast track evidence-based herbal drug development following Reverse Pharmacology path. Phytomics, a technology platform for characterization of herbal compositions wherein, Herbal Bio Response Arrays (HBR Arrays) are used to determine bioactive constituents and biological activities of an herbal composition has recently been developed and patented.

Further, CAM disciplines owing to their holistic nature may be impacting gene expression and signaling pathways. Application of such novel expression analysis tools may help to understand and characterize the genes and signaling pathways involved in CAM modalities.

DNA microarrays have the potential for application in different phases of herbal drug discovery and development. This includes quality control and standardization of the herbal drugs, identification and validation of new targets, the profiling of on-target and off-target effects during the optimization of new therapeutic agents, understanding molecular mechanisms of action, structure-activity relationships and the prediction of side-effects, and the discovery of diagnostic, prognostic, and pharmacodynamic bio-markers.

At present the major practical applicability of DNA microarrays remains in SNP mapping, genotyping and pharmacogenetics. In recent years, array-based sequencing (minisequencing/resequencing arrays) that combines target hybridization with enzymatic primer extension reactions has emerged as a powerful means to scan for all possible DNA sequence variations.

Highly multiplexed microarray systems offering potential for mutation analysis and genome-wide SNP mapping have been developed. DNA microarrays are a effective new strategy for global gene expression profiling, but reliable detection of expression changes and understanding the functional relevance of these expression profiles is a challenge. Other problems in microarray experiments include non-reproducibility, difficulty in statistical analysis and comparability of data from different experiments.

Inconsistencies in data may arise due to low specificity of cDNA probes, discrepancy in fold-change calculations, variations in laboratories, technicians, probe labeling, biochemical reactions, scanners, lasers etc. Also the sensitivity and specificity of DNA microarrays depends on the nucleotide composition of the target and probe. Repetitive sequence elements and highly structured nucleic acids can greatly decrease the sensitivity of hybridization based analysis.

In its current stage, a microarray experiment needs to be validated by independent confirmation of results by laboratory-based analysis and in silico comparison with information available in literature and expression databases. Although DNA microarrays have huge potential for pharmacodynamics and toxigenomics applications, these are still in exploratory stage and need validation by other biological experiments. Bio-informatics and statistical tools have a major role to play in the microarray field, whereby data from multiple experiments can be integrated to answer complex biological questions.

Another factor limiting microarray application is the cost of the technology. The challenge today is to provide standardized, sensitive, reproducible microarray platforms, databases and visualization methods for expression profiles that are also affordable to scientists. With the development of new, uniform and more sophisticated experimental designs, data management systems statistical tools and algorithms for data analysis DNA microarrays can be optimally used in herbal drug research.

In spite of the huge potential offered by microarray technology, the importance of in vitro biological assays, cell-line studies and in vivo animal studies cannot be ignored. A comprehensive strategy integrating information from diverse scientific experiments and technologies will lead to molecular evidence-based herbal medicine.

6

Guidelines for Medicinal Plants

The guidelines for "Good Agricultural Practice of Medicinal and Aromatic Plants" are intended to apply to the growing and primary processing of all such plants as traded and used in the European Union. Hence, they apply to the production of all plant materials used in the food, feed, medicinal, flavouring and perfumery industries.

They also apply to all methods of production including organic production in accordance with the European Union regulations. Those farmers involved in the production of medicinal and aromatic plants should ensure that damage to the existing wildlife habitats is avoided and that efforts are made to maintain and enhance the biodiversity of their farms. It is advisable to regulate wild gathering by a specific guideline.

The present Good Agricultural Practice guidelines provide additional standards for the production and processing of raw materials insofar as they mainly focus on identifying those critical production measures that are necessary in contributing to good product quality.

In this respect, an attempt will be made to minimize insufficient quality by prevention means. The main aim of GAP guidelines is to ensure that the plant raw material meets the demands of the consumer and thus fulfils high quality standards. It is therefore important that they:

- Are produced hygienically, in order to reduce microbiological load to a minimum,

- Are produced with care, so that negative effect on plants in the course of cultivation, processing and storage is limited.

Since medicinal and aromatic plants and their products are exposed to a large number of microbiological and other contaminants in the course of the production process, the main aim of the present guidelines is to provide guidance for producers to reduce this plant raw material contamination to the lowest possible minimum.

All participants in the production process (from primary producers to traders) are required to comply with these guidelines voluntarily and to develop practical measures in order to realize them.

Producers, traders and processors of medicinal and aromatic plants, especially of tea-related and herbal medicinal products, should comply with the GAP guidelines, document their products by a way bill (batch documentation) and demand that their partners also adhere to these requirements.

Guidelines for Good Agricultural Practice

Seeds and Propagation Material

Seeds in use are to be identified botanically, indicating plant variety, cultivar, chemotype and origin. The material used should be 100 % traceable. The same applies to vegetatively propagated parent material. Parent material used in organic production has to be certified as authentically organic.

The parent material should meet the requirements/ standards concerning purity and germination (where available: certified seed/propagation material should be used). The parent material should be as free as possible from pests and diseases in order to guarantee healthy plant growth. If resistant or tolerant species or origins are available, they should be preferred.

The occurrence of plants and plant parts that are not species/ variety identical has to be controlled in the course of the entire production process (cultivation, harvest, drying, packaging). Any impurites have to be eliminated promptly. Plant materials or seeds derived from or comprising genetically modified organsims have to comply with national and European Union regulations.

Cultivation

Depending on the method of cultivation *e.g.* conventional or organic, growers should be allowed to follow different "Standard Operating Procedures" for cultivation (to be elaborated). In general, care should be taken to avoid environmental disturbances. The principles of good crop husbandry must be followed including an appropriate rotation of crops.

Soil and Fertilization

Medicinal and aromatic plants should not be grown in soils that are contaminated by sludge. Furthermore, soils should not be contaminated by heavy metals, residues of plant protection products and any other unnatural chemicals. It should therefore be endeavoured to apply the use of chemical products with as minimum negative effect as possible.

The manure applied should be void of human faeces and be thoroughly composted prior to application. All other fertilizing agents should be applied sparingly and in accordance with the demands of the plant and the particular species (including application between harvests). The use of fertilizers should be in accordance with efforts to minimize leaching.

Irrigation

Irrigation should be minimized as much as possible and only be applied according to the needs of the plant.

Water used for irrigation should comply with national and European Union quality standards and be as free as possible from contaminants, such as faeces, heavy metals, pesticides, herbicides and toxicologically hazardous substances.

Crop Maintenance and Plant Protection

Tillage should be adapted to the growth and requirements of plants. Pesticide and herbicide application should be avoided as far as possible. When necessary, they should be carried out using the minimum effective rates of approved plant protection products. Products for chemical plant protection have to conform with the European Union's maximum residue limits (European Pharmacopoeia, European Directives, Codex Alimentarius). Application and storage of plant protection products have to be in conformity with the regulations of manufacturers and the respective national authorities.

The application should only be carried out by qualified staff using approved equipment. Application should precede the harvest by a period either defined by the buyer or indicated by the producer of the plant protection product.

The use of pesticides and herbicides has to be documented.

All measures regarding nutrient supply and chemical plant protection, should secure the marketability of the product. It is obligatory that the buyer of the batch be informed of the brand, quantity and date of pesticide use in written form.

Harvest

Harvesting should take place when the plants are of best possible quality, according to their different utilizations.

Harvesting should preferably take place under the best possible conditions (wet soils, dew, rain or exceptionally high air humidity can be unfavourable). If harvesting is done under wet conditions, extra care should be taken in order to avoid the unfavourable influence of moisture.

Equipment should be kept in clean and technically perfect working condition. Those machine parts, including their housing, that have direct contact with the harvested crop should be regularly cleaned and kept free of oil and other contaminants (including plant left-overs).

Cutting devices of harvesters must be adjusted so that their collection of soil particles is reduced to a minimum.

In the course of harvesting, care should be taken to ensure that no toxic weeds are mixed with the harvested crop.

Damaged and perished plant parts must be promptly sorted out.

All containers used in the harvest must be cleaned and kept free of the remnants of previous crops; containers not in use, must also be preserved in a dry condition, free of pests and inaccessible to mice/rodents as well as livestock and other domestic animals.

The harvested crop should not come into direct contact with the soil. It must be promptly collected and submitted to transport under dry and clean conditions (by use of sacks, baskets, trailers, containers, etc.).

Mechanical damage and compacting of the crop that may result in undesirable quality changes must be avoided. In this respect, attention must be paid in ensuring that:

- The sacks are not overfilled,
- The stacking up of sacks does not result in thickening of the crop,
- The harvested crop is transported and kept in containers or bags in such a way that the occurence of heating up is prevented.

Delivery of freshly harvested plant material to the processing facility must occur as quickly as possible in order to prevent its heating up.

The harvested crop must be protected from pests, mice/ rodents and domestic animals. Pest control measures should be documented.

Primary Processing

Primary processing after harvest includes such processing steps as washing, freezing, distilling, drying, etc. All these processes, whether for food or medicinal use, must conform to European Union and other national regulations.

On arrival at the processing facility, the harvested crop has to be promptly unloaded and unpacked. Prior to processing the material should not be directly exposed to the sun (except where there is specific need *e.g.* distillation) and it must be protected from rainfall.

Buildings used in the processing of harvested crops must be clean, thoroughly aerated and should not be used for the housing of livestock. Buildings should be so constructed as to provide protection for the harvested crop against birds, insects, rodents as well as domestic animals. In all storage (including packaging) and processing areas, suitable pest control measures, such as baits and electric insect killing machines, must be operated and maintained by professionally qualified staff or contractors.

Processing equipment must be kept clean and be regularly serviced.

In the case of natural open air drying, the crop must be spread out in a thin layer. In order to secure unlimited air circulation, the drying frames must be located at a sufficient distance above the ground. Attempts must be made to achieve uniform drying of the crop so as to avoid mould formation.

When drying with oil, the exhaust fumes should not be reused for drying. Direct drying should not be allowed except with butane, propane, or natural gas.

Except in the case of natural open air drying, the conditions (*e.g.* temperature, duration, etc.) must be selected taking into consideration the type (*e.g.* root, leaf or flower) and active substance content (*e.g.* essential oils and others) of the crude drug to be produced.

Drying conditions should be documented.

Drying directly on the ground with direct exposure to sunlight should be avoided unless it is required for a particular plant.

All material must be sorted or sieved in order to eliminate sub-standard products and foreign bodies. Sieves must be maintained in a clean state and should be serviced regularly.

Clearly marked waste-bins should be kept handy, emptied and cleaned daily.

The dried product should be promptly packaged in order to protect it from and reduce the risk of pest attacks.

Packaging

After the repeated control and eventual elimination of low-quality materials and any foreign bodies, the product should be preferably packaged in new, clean and dry sacks, bags or chests. The label must be clear, permanently fixed and be made of non-toxic material. Information must conform with the European Union and national labelling regulations.

Packaging materials should be stored in a clean and dry place that is free of pests and inaccessible to livestock and other domestic animals. It must be guaranteed that no product contamination occurs as a result of using packaging material, particularly in the case of fibre bags.

Reusable packaging materials should be well cleaned and perfectly dried prior to their usage. It must be guaranteed that no contamination takes place by reusing bags.

Storage and Transport

Packaged dried materials and essential oils should be stored in a dry, well aerated building, in which the daily temperature fluctuations are limited and good aeration is guaranteed. Fresh products (except basil) should be stored between 1°C and 5°C while frozen products should be stored below -18°C (or below -20°C for longer term storage).

Essential oil storage must conform to the appropriate chemical storage standards.

As a protection against pests, birds, rodents and domestic animals, the window and door openings should be protected, *e.g.* by wire netting.

It is recommended that the packaged dry crop be stored as follows:

- In buildings with concrete or similar easily cleanable floors,
- On pallets,
- With sufficient distance from the wall,
- With thorough separation from other crops to avoid cross-contamination
- And organic products must be stored separately.

In case of bulk delivery, it is important to ensure that the transportation conditions are dry. Furthermore, it is highly advisable to use aerated containers in order to reduce the risk of mould formation or fermentation. As a supplement, the use of other sufficiently aerated transport vehicles and other aerated facilities is recommended. Essential oil transportation must conform to the relevant and applicable regulations. In this respect, national and European Union regulations on transport have to be adhered to.

Fumigation against pest attack should only be carried out on necessity and must exclusively be administered by licensed personnel. Only registered chemicals should be used. Any fumigation against pest attack should be reported in the documentation.

For fumigation of warehouses, only permitted substances should be used in accordance with European Union or national regulations.

Whenever frozen storage or saturated steam is used for pest control, the humidity of the stored material must be controlled after each treatment.

Equipment

Equipment used in plant cultivation and processing should be easy to clean, in order to eliminate the risk of contamination.

All machinery should be mounted in an easily accessible position. They must be well serviced and cleaned regularly. Fertilizer and pesticide application machinery must be regularly calibrated.

Preferably, non-wooden equipment should be used unless tradition requires the use of wooden material. Whenever wooden equipment is used (*e.g.* pallets, racks, bunkers, etc.), care should be taken to avoid its direct contact with chemical and other contaminated/infected materials, so as to prevent the impurity of the plant material.

Personnel and Facilities

Personnel should receive adequate botanical education before performing tasks that require this knowledge.

All processing procedures should fully conform with both EU-guidelines on food hygiene and the general food hygienic principles of Codex Alimentarius as well as the European directive on Good Manufacturing Practice (GMP).

The personnel entrusted with the handling of plant material are required to exhibit a high degree of personal hygiene (including those personnel working in the fields) and should have received adequate training in their hygienic responsibilities.

The buildings where the plant processing is carried out have to be equipped with changing facilities as well as toilets and hand washing facilities, with respect to the relevant regulations. Persons suffering from known infectious diseases transmittable via food, including diarrhoea, or being transmitters of such diseases, must be denied entry into areas where they may come into contact with the plant material, as per relevant regulations.

Persons with open wounds, inflammations and skin infections should be kept away from those areas where plant processing takes place, or have to wear appropriate protective clothing or gloves, until their complete recuperation.

Personnel should be protected from contact with toxic or potentially allergenic plant materials by means of adequate protective clothing.

The welfare of all staff involved in the growing and processing of medicinal and aromatic plant products should be ensured.

Documentation

All parent materials and processing steps, including the location of cultivation, have to be documented. Field records showing previous cropping and used inputs should be maintained by all growers.

All batches from coherent areas should be clearly and unmistakably labelled (*e.g.* by the application of a batch number). This should take place as early as possible.

Batches from different cultivation areas may be mixed only if it is guaranteed that the mixture in itself will be homogenous. Such mixing procedures should also be documented.

It is essential to document the type, quantity and date of harvest of the crop, as well as the chemicals and other substances (*e.g.* fertilizers, pesticides and herbicides, growth regulators, etc.) used during production.

The application of fumigation agents such as phosphin must be entered into batch documentation.

All processes and procedures that could bear any impact on the quality of the product must be entered into the batch documentation.

All agreements (production guidelines, contracts, etc.) between the producer and the buyer should be laid down in written form.

It should be documented in a way bill (batch documentation) that cultivation, harvesting and production have been performed in accordance with the GAP guidelines. Minimal information included in the way bill should cover the geographical definition of growth place, the country of origin and the responsible producer.

Audit results should be documented in an audit report (*i.e.* copies of all documents, reference index, audit reports, analysis results) and be stored for a minimum of 10 years.

Any special circumstances during the growth period which may influence the chemical composition, *e.g.* extreme weather conditions or pests - particularly in the harvest period - must be documented.

Education

It is highly advisable to educate all personnel dealing with the crop or those engaged in the management of production, in production techniques as well as the appropriate use of herbicides and pesticides.

Quality Guarantee

Consultation between producers and buyers of medicinal and aromatic plants, with regard to quality questions, *e.g.* active principles and other characteristic ingredients, optical and sensoric properties, limited germ numbers, plant protection chemical residues and heavy metals, must be based on nternationally recognized or national specifications and should be laid down in written form.

Medicinal Plants

The American public has a longtime love affair with herbs. A few years ago everyone was grinding basil for pesto, stuffing rosemary in their vinegar bottles, and putting French tarragon sprigs on their chicken. Then they moved on to herbal wreathes, soaps, and potpourris. Now companies across the nation indicate that herbal medicines and aromatherapy are the fastest growing sales categories. The general feeling in the industry is that the public's interest in herbs has not reached its peak and healthy growth is expected in the future.

So what can that mean for you as a propagator? Retail nurseries report that gardeners are very interested in growing their own medicinal herb plants. People are in the market for shade loving perennials, such as ginseng and goldenseal; sun-loving plants, such as purple coneflower; and shrubs and trees, such as witch hazel and ginkgo.

The companies producing medicinal herb products, such as the capsules and tinctures you find in health food stores and pharmacies, have traditionally purchased most of their raw herbs from India, China, and the Eastern European countries. As the medicinal herb industry has matured, however, the companies buying these herbs have instituted new quality control efforts that include testing for active compounds, purity, and bacterial contamination. Many companies have found that foreign imports do not meet their new high standards.

This has opened up a market for American growers to produce large acreages of medicinal herbs. This, in turn, has created a market for the seeds and plants to produce these herbs. That is where you as a propagator can get involved with herbs. So let me tell you about some of the plants that are currently in demand and some of what is known about producing these plants.

There are several important points to keep in mind before you jump into medicinal plant production. One is that you are working with "new crops". Thus, your county extension office will not have information packed bulletins on how to grow most of these plants. I encourage you to read everything you can about the herb plants we do know something about, and about plants that are similar to what you want to grow. Talk to the people at your local botanical garden and to herb enthusiasts. Mostly, you must rely on your own experience, horticultural knowledge, and "gut instincts." Keep careful notes on everything you do and the results you obtain. You could quickly find yourself the expert on propagation of one of these little known medicinal herbs.

Second, be very careful about where you buy your seeds and planting stock. This is a new industry and quality standards aren't always what they should be. Check your sources out very carefully. If you decide to collect seeds and planting stock from wild populations, be certain to check on local regulations and the status of plants before you head out. Some of the more popular medicinal herbs are endangered or protected species in some states.

For any of the shade-loving plants, of course, you must provide shade. Commercial herb growers use natural shade or artificial shade provided by wood lath or polypropylene shade cloth. When using artificial shade, I recommend tall structures, about 8-9 feet tall, with two open ends for good ventilation.

What are some of the plants in demand? Right now, one of the plants in greatest demand is goldenseal; Hydrastis canadensis, a shade loving, herbaceous perennial. It is used for many purposes including as a treatment for AIDS, cancer, various digestive disorders, and to boost the immune system. It is native to North America and used to grow in abundance throughout the Appalachian region. Unfortunately, native populations have been seriously reduced by over collection and it is now an endangered species in North Carolina and under new regulations for international trade.

Goldenseal has a rhizome by which it spreads rapidly and is easily propagated. In fall or spring, these rhizomes can be cut into pieces. Try to include an obvious bud on each piece, but research indicates that it is even more important to have good roots. Goldenseal produces a raspberry like fruit, which is full of seeds. These seed require special handling, such as they cannot be allowed to dry out. Most growers find they get the best germination when the seed are sown immediately after they are extracted from the fruit. This, of course, is not real practical for the propagator.

Studies are underway at North Carolina Statue University looking at seed extraction methods, seed disinfection treatments, seed storage temperature regimes, and planting dates. So far, the best germination has been obtained from seed that had been held at 70 degrees F prior to sowing in late August or late October.

Studies are also being conducted on soil fertility, mulch, and spacing for goldenseal. For the fertility studies, goldenseal was grown for three years in forest soil amended to provide four levels of lime, phosphorus, and nitrogen. Emergence the first year was greatly influenced by lime application. Emergence was very low where the soil pH was lower than 4.8 or higher than 6.7. If the plants made it through that first year at the undesirable pH levels, they exhibited 90% or better germination the following years. Any supplemental nitrogen, reduced emergence that first year, but had little effect in the following years. The response to phosphate, supplied as superphosphate, was much the same. As with emergence, the plants were tallest around pH 5.5 and 6.5.

Goldenseal roots and rhizomes are the plant parts of interest to the propagators and the botanical ingredient companies. There was a dramatic response in growth of these parts to soil pH. The bottom line is, remember to keep pH around 5.5 to 6.5. These numbers will be refined as further research is conducted. Fresh root weight was inversely related to increasing nitrogen rate during the first year of growth. There were no significant responses to nitrogen rate after the second or third year, however. The response to phosphate additions was very similar.

Studies are now underway looking at spacing effects. Plants emerged first in the closest spacings of 2x2 inches and 4x4 inches. Mulch studies were also initiated in 1997. Plants grew best the first season with bark mulches, pine needles, and sawdust. Straw mulch resulted in poor growth and severe slug damage. Shade requirements are also being examined with plants growing under polypropylene shade providing 30%, 47%, 63%, 80% shade and wood lath.

So, as you can see—there was a lot we didn't know, and still don't know, about growing goldenseal. However, for those willing to try and work out the cultivation methods, there are good markets for goldenseal seedlings and mature plants for planting stock. There also is a limited, but growing market, for goldenseal plants for retail sales.

American ginseng (Panax quinquefolium) is another medicinal herb that has a long history of cultivation in North America. You will have no problem finding information on ginseng seed handling and plant growing. Ginseng seed requires very special handling and a stratification period of about 18 months. Like goldenseal, ginseng seed must never be allowed to dry out. There are a large number of suppliers of ginseng seed and roots for commercial growers. However, there are few nurseries catering to the home gardeners. A few enterprising growers have tapped into this lucrative hobbyist market. These plants sell for $12 to $25 a piece.

Other shade requiring medicinal plants in demand include black cohosh (Cimicufuga racemosa)—a perennial shrub, fairly easy to propagate by root division or seed. The roots of this plant are used to treat various feminine disorders. Mayapple (Podophyllum peltatum) is another woodland plant in demand because of its cancer fighting properties.

It is propagated primarily by dividing the roots in the spring because the seeds can be hard to germinate. The plant thrives, however, under cultivation. Bloodroot (Sanguinaria canadensis) has a pretty, early spring flower which makes this plant especially attractive to the retail market. Bloodroot can be easily propagated by seed or root division. Bloodroot is used in a popular toothpaste because of its antiplaque properties. It also has other antibacterial properties. It can be quite toxic, however, at low doses!

Chamelirium luteum goes by many common names, including fairy wand, star grub root, Helonias, and devil's bit. The plant is an erect, fleshy, perennial with a rosette of leaves at the base. Male and female flowers are borne on separate plants. This plant has not really been cultivated and we know little about its requirements. However, demand for this plant is increasing. The roots are used to treat a variety of feminine disorders. Any herb that can be of use to the aging baby boomers, especially to help them deal with problems related to menopause, prostate, poor memory, and low energy, will have a strong market!

A sunloving, field grown plant that does well for plant sales include all the different species of Echinacea, including angustifolia, purpurea, and pallida. The most common use for Echinacea right now is to help boost the immune system to prevent catching colds and the flu. Skullcap (Scutellaria lateriflora) is in demand as transplants for a field crop. It is easily grown from seeds. Skullcap is used as a sedative and to treat headaches. Calendula (Calendula officinalia) is a very attractive herb, commonly used in home herb gardens but also grown in large acreages. It is easily grown from seed. Calendula is valued for its wound healing properties.

If you decide that you want to get into the medicinal herb plant business, you need to know what is happening in the industry. My first recommendation is that you subscribe to some of the more popular herb publications. The demand for various herbs can change rapidly, and it is important to keep abreast of what is happening in the industry. For information on the industry in general, with emphasis on retail, look at publications such as the "Business of Herbs" and the "Herbal Connection". Information of this sort on the wholesale and field grown medicinals is harder to come by, but "HerbalGram" and the trade publications for natural foods are good places to start.

"ATTRAnews," the newsletter from the federally funded programme called Appropriate Technology Transfer for Rural Areas, is a publication that is useful to anyone looking at commercial production of alternative crops.

Some of the companies buying herbs and contract growing also can provide some useful production information. And some seed companies who sell large volumes of herb seed provide technical assistance. For example, Johnny's Selected Seeds hired medicinal plant experts as consultants to help with their herb line and Richter's Herb Seeds holds a growers conference every year. I also recommend that you join local and national herb associations. For example, the International Herb Association provides good networking opportunities, holds a national conference each year, and has regional chapters that can be a good source of information.

Currently the market is strong for medicinal herbs so many growers are jumping into it. But the ones that stay with it and find it profitable will be the ones who do their homework, grow a quality plant, and provide the service and prices the market demands.

Medicinal Plants of Meru

Since ancient times, Meru people in Kenya have largely depended on their local plants for medicines, food, fuels, material and environmental uses including hedges, shades, and land markers. Meru bee plants are used in beehive smoking and bee attractors, while other plants for social use include masticatories and those used in games and in smoking. Traditional cosmetic and aromatic plants are used for Meru socio-cultural puroposes. In the ethnobotanical study conducted in Meru (Kenya) in 2002 and 2003 was found that Meru people know and use over 635 different species of plants for the various needs listed above. Of the total number of 635, not less than 411 were medicinal plants, while a few were cosmetic and aromatic plants. The study has documented the indigenous plant classification, local use and management practices, and related illnesses.

Medicinal Plants in Health

Various trees, shrubs, herbs, climbers and creepers/climbers, grass, succulents, bulbs and rhizomes are mainly used to prepare traditional medicines. The specific parts of the plant that make the medicines include bark, roots (tuber), leaves and buds. The preparation of herbal medicine varies for 'external' and' internal' illnesses.

A large number of perceived diseases have been reported to be mainly treated through the application of specific traditional herbal medicine. These include: head, tooth and gum aches, sore eyes, growths on the face, common colds, and dandruffs, brain fatigue, tonsillitis, mumps, mouth sores and aching ears. Also, neck stiffness, asthma, coughs, chest pains, pneumonia, tuberculosis, and whooping cough belong to this category of diseases.

Stomach ailments treated by herbal medicine include acidity, ulcers, worms, heartburn, diarrhoea, constipation, amoeba, poisons, anthrax, nausea and cholera. Backaches, joint aches, swollen legs, sprains and rheumatism are also among the diseases treated by traditional plant-based medicines. Special herbal remedies are reported for malaria and other kinds of fevers, rashes, boils, measles, itching, scurvy, skin growths, dry skin and ringworms. Similarly, venereal diseases, fresh cuts, wounds from poisoned arrows, burns, anaemia, diabetes and high blood pressure are mostly treated by traditional herbal medicines.

Antenatal herbal treatment include birth control; abortifecients and menstrual overflow while post-natal treatments include problems related to afterbirths and excessive bleeding.

Medicinal Plants in Culture

Plants in Meru have been part of the local people's culture for as long as they have known them. There are particular trees that are believed to give long life - the Mugumo tree; those that give healing by just singing praises to them (Mutuntu) and those that bring prosperity and health to couples and families (Kirao).

Cultural diversity is also manifest in Meru people views on herbal medicines. The differential perceptions are influenced by a variety of factors. These include socio-demographic *e.g.* ethnicity, religion; psyco-social *e.g.* knowledge, attitudes and beliefs; and enabling factors *e.g.* socio-economic status and profession of respondents.

Cosmetic and Aromatic Plants in Health and Culture

Although fewer people tend to use plant-based products nowadays due to the already available cosmetic and aromatic products found at modern chemists, there is recently a reorientation towards the use of cosmetic plants. Some parts of Kenya still use wild plants for their cosmetic products, but the Meru people only knows these specific plants from the past.

The main reported uses then include traditional perfumes for circumcised girls and women. Among young children, particular roots of cosmetic plants are crushed and the powder mixed with saliva and applied on the body of a child, also to cure colds and coughs. An example of such a plant is the Ndago plant.

Medicinal Plants—Industrial Profiles

Which well known plant never touches the ground, does not follow a 12-month vegetation cycle, stays green year round, blooms in the winter, and sells predominately in December? The answer, of course, is mistletoe. Current research questions the efficacy of this highly controversial plant. "Rejected by clinical oncologists but used by practitioners and cancer patients, it is applied as a remedy to treat a broad spectrum of different diseases, such as epilepsy, diabetes, hypertension, arthrosis, hepatitis, HIV infection, labour pains, and cancer."

Now a new book on the therapeutic uses and industrial applications of Viscum has been published. Rarely mentioned in traditional books on herbal medicine mistletoe research remains questionable. Because the "extracts may exert different effects than purified substances" individual immune responses vary greatly. There is a great need for further investigation. Currently no clinical data are available documenting long-term therapy treatment.

Whether the extracts of Viscum become a major player in the fight against cancer, this book makes for provocative reading. Researchers in pharmacognosy and phystochemistry will find this book documented with references to hundreds of research articles invaluable. While most articles feature the European point of view, there is one article from Japan and another from South Africa. Although none of the articles originate from the United States, American research is well represented in the bibliographies, as are traditional Chinese uses for this herb.

Responding to the increased demand for information on medicinal and aromatic plants this fascinating look at this highly controversial plant is the 16th volume in the series Medicinal and Aromatic Plants Industrial Profiles. This series brings together articles scattered through a variety of sources, is international in scope, and includes many little known sources. Each article is well documented and is introduced by the editor Arndt Bussing, head of the Department of Applied Immunology at the foundation Krebsforschung Herdecke, University of Witten/Herdecke. Mistletoe: the Genus Viscum is illustrated with colour photographs of the plant, line drawings, and chemical structures. With few exceptions most references are current, dating from 1990 to 2000.

While this book would be of interest to scientists in botany, agriculture, and phytochemistry, those working in alternative medicine, pharmaceutical, and health sciences should find it of greater interest. Recommended for academic and research libraries.

New Support for Medicinal Plants

Aspirin, ginseng tea, Aloe lotions and gels are simple healthcare remedies used in many parts of the world to treat a variety of illnesses. They all also have a common beginning: wild plants. Aspirin, for instance, owes its origins to the willow tree.

Hippocrates used powder extracted from willow bark to treat pain and reduce fever in the fifth century BC. Over 2000 years later, the chemical compound salicin was isolated from willow bark, the precursor to the active compound found in modern aspirin. Today, it is estimated that more than 80 billion aspirin tablets are used each year in the USA alone. Unlike aspirin, ginseng tea, used to improve vital energy and slow aging, is still produced from the raw product: ginseng roots. However, much of the ginseng in trade is cultivated, as is all of the aloe vera gel found in skin-care products and health drinks.

Less well known are the tens and perhaps hundreds of thousands of other medicinal plant species used around the world, some of which, like willow trees, have been recognised for their healing properties for thousands of years.

These plants form the basis of health care systems throughout much of the developing world, a source of new compounds on which to base new pharmaceutical products, and a major component of the burgeoning markets for herbal health care remedies and natural products. They also provide a source of income for growers, traders, collectors and manufacturers of plant-based medicines.

In this dual role as a source of healthcare and income, medicinal plants make an important contribution to the larger development process. Unfortunately, however, some plant species of medicinal value are already in short supply, which poses a threat to human welfare and the wild species themselves. Immediate actions are therefore required to ensure harvest and trade of medicinal plant species are conducted sustainably.

TRAFFIC has been working on the medicinal plant trade for many years, including collaboration with important partners such as the IUCN/SSC Medicinal Plant Specialist Group.

Germany's Federal Ministry for Economic Cooperation and Development (Bundesministerium fur wirtschaftliche Zusammenarbeit, more commonly known as BMZ) is supporting a suite of new actions by TRAFFIC. Through a Funds in Trust Agreement with WWF International, BMZ has pledged DM1 million (US$560 000) to the TRAFFIC Network's medicinal plant work during 1998-2000. Much of the funding is directed toward regionally focused work in East Asia, the Indian subcontinent and South America.

In addition, BMZ is supporting efforts to build and/or strengthen links with others working on medicinal plant trade issues. It aims to enhance the communication of TRAFFIC's research results to those who need it, from traditional medicine communities to policy makers.

The regional work to be undertaken through BMZ support is as diverse as the medicinal plant trade itself, with each region home to different, but in the case of India and East Asia, overlapping, medicinal traditions.

East Asia

The major traditional medicine systems in this region are derived from traditional Chinese medicine (TCM), which has a history of several thousand years and is well-documented.

Although international attention has been drawn to the use of animal species such as rhinoceros and Tiger in TCM, animal ingredients actually make up less than 20% of those used in TCM. TCM is largely a plant-based medicinal system. It is believed that as many as 1000 plant species are in use for TCM in China and that about 80 per cent of them are taken from the wild. An initial TRAFFIC East Asia study in Hong Kong in 1995/96 revealed a massive trade involving a number of threatened plant species: of the 388 plant species listed in the China Plant Red Data Book, 69 were found to be used in TCM, and 22 of these were in common use.

Through work supported by BMZ, TRAFFIC East Asia seeks to promote the security and conservation of wild plant resources used in traditional medicine in East Asia to support basic health care needs.

TRAFFIC East Asia will convene a series of meetings to promote dialogue and understanding of the links between conservation and medicinal security issues among producers, regulators and medicinal communities.

Other activities planned include the compilation of an overview of the nature of and trends in medicinal plant harvest, propagation and trade in East Asia; identifying species at risk; and reviewing national legislation and policies relevant to production, supply and conservation of medicinal plants. Work will also be undertaken to help build capacity within governments and TCM communities to implement any needed trade controls.

The Indian subcontinent

The Himalayas provide more than a meeting point for China and the Indian subcontinent. They also provide a huge variety and volume of medicinal plants used in TCM, Tibetan medicine, and Ayurved. Like TCM, Ayurved has a long history (over 3000 years), is well-documented, and is widely used both locally and in Asian communities established in other parts of the world. There are also a large number of localised traditional medicine systems.

Harvest of native plants to supply India's own healthcare needs and a growing export market provides an important source of income for local communities. However, demand for plant materials is huge and growing, while many of the region's medicinal plant resources are dwindling. Recent reviews applying IUCN threat criteria found that a significant number of medicinal plant species are threatened or endangered within India. Large quantities of raw medicinal plant materials are also imported into India from neighbouring countries and exported to overseas markets.

A number of organizations within India are concerned with maintaining India's traditional medicine systems. In addition, there is a widespread development network, an established pharmaceutical industry and a wealth of botanical experts in the country. Until now, however, there has been little effort to document the volume and impact of national or international trade in India's medicinal plants.

TRAFFIC India is already well on its way toward establishing working relationships with key stake-holders such as those above and government personnel and toward collecting information required if plants in trade are to be managed on a sustainable basis.

A key challenge within India will be to inform these and other stake-holders of the nature and impact of the medicinal plant trade, and to facilitate their co-operation in developing and implementing measures that will secure the conservation of medicinal plants. Original research will be combined with meetings and workshops to discuss findings and develop workable solutions to any problems identified.

South America

In contrast to East Asia and India, South America's traditional medicine practices are far more localised, with neither the geographic extent or the written texts that characterise TCM and Ayurved. As a result, an important first step is to study and describe the medicinal plant trade in the region, to identify commonly used species, and to begin the process of identifying whether any species are at risk.

Preliminary research in 1996 and 1997 by TRAFFIC International's South America Plants Officer confirmed that, as in Asia, medicinal plants are important components of local health care, are in some cases used unsustainably, and are exported as well as used locally.

BMZ funding is supporting the completion of a regional overview of the medicinal plant trade as well as more detailed studies of individual species in trade, existing trade controls, and the potential role of regional and international treaties in this region. Two species already identified for further research are Cat's Claw Uncaria tomentosa and Dragon's Blood Croton lechleri.

The results of this research will be shared with governments, traditional healthcare associations and relevant agencies to further raise the profile of medicinal plant trade issues and stimulate discussion and actions necessary to ensure more effective management.

Medicinal Plants and CITES

The Challenge of Sustainable Harvest

Plants of medicinal value originate from all over the world. Harvest occurs for both local and international use. A growing problem, which is compounded by global population growth and increased demand for raw materials, is over-exploitation of these important resources. The vast majority of medicinal plants used in traditional medical systems and natural products industries are collected from the wild. While propagation occurs for a few species such as American Ginseng Panax quinquefolius and Kuth Saussurea costus, propagation is generally limited due to the expense and time periods required for plants to reach salable size. Harvest and trade can be an important source of income for rural peoples. Regrettably, unsustainable harvest is an increasingly common occurrence that threatens not only the future of these species, but also the livelihoods and health status of people throughout the world.

The Current Situation

At present an estimated 230 plant species included in CITES are traded for medicinal purposes, or are likely to be traded in the future. Fourteen of these were specifically included in the Appendices expressly because of the need to regulate trade in medicinal material. A further six species, Adonis vernalis, Camptotheca acuminata, Cistanche deserticola, Harpagophytum procumbens, Harpagophytum zeyheri and Panax ginseng, are proposed for inclusion in Appendix II at COP11.

The Parties' implementation of the Convention for the species currently included in the Appendices is poor, and is in many cases non-existent. This is surprising, given the importance of these species to the health care of the peoples of these nations, to the livelihoods of the millions who derive income from medicinal plant harvest and trade, and to the industries and consumers who benefit from these resources. Indeed, some Parties have made notable efforts to implement CITES for medicinal plants, such as Germany with the publication of the Checklist of Medicinal and Aromatic Plants and their Trade Names covered by CITES and EU Regulation 2307/97 and Identification Training for Medicinal and Aromatic Plants covered by CITES and EU Regulation 2307/97, and USA with the establishment of a ginseng management programme to monitor wild populations and regulate harvest and commerce.

The Plants Committee has examined the trade through the Medicinal Plant Significant Trade Study, and additional significant plant trade surveys have been undertaken by TRAFFIC. However, these efforts are few in number and although Parties may have taken domestic measures to conserve native plant populations, in general, implementation of the Convention for medicinal plants is unsatisfactory.

Over-exploitation of medicinal plants, and lack of attention to illegal and unsustainable trade, is having serious repercussions around the world. As the global population expands, the demand for medicine increases correspondingly. International trade in medicinal and aromatic plants is already massive, with for example, annual global market imports totalling 440,000 metric tonnes in 1996, at a value of USD

1.3 billion. The medicinal plant trade can make a considerable contribution to the economies of producer countries.

Searching for Solutions

As medicinal plant populations decline, governments, natural resource managers, local communities and a variety of other stake-holders have attempted to address the problem in order to conserve medicinal resources. Efforts have been varied.

For example, these initiatives include: promotion of sustainable harvesting techniques; improvement of marketing and trade opportunities to ensure better management; training in quality control and packaging to reduce wastage and derive higher earnings; increased regulation and control at local, national and international levels; and propagation of medicinal plant species. Increasingly, these efforts are designed taking into consideration the complexity of the medicinal plant issue and the realization that demand will not decrease, hence solutions must factor in the aspect of a continuously increasing trade.

The market for medicinal plants is dynamic and complex. Demand for new natural products, and growing interest in traditional medical systems around the world, means that greater volumes of plant material are required to satisfy the market. Medicinal plants are traded in a variety of forms, for example: raw material such as leaves, bark, and roots, unprocessed broken material such as chips or slices, derivatives and semi-processed or manufactured material such as powders, extracts, tonics, pills, teas and other products, as well as finished pharmaceutical products.

Trade occurs far from the area of production, and processing often takes place in countries other than those where the plants originate. For example, approximately 120,000 metric tonnes of medicinal and aromatic plants were imported into Europe in 1996, and this material came from over 120 countries, 60% of which were African and Asian nations. During this same year, Europe exported about 70,000 metric tonnes of plant material. Understanding the dynamics of the trade in medicinals can be difficult, and although overall volumes and values may be known, species-specific information is not at all comprehensive. The dearth of such data is one reason for the lack of attention countries have directed toward the medicinal plant resource.

Insufficient knowledge about the scope of the trade, in particular at the range state level, has resulted in ineffective implementation of existing regulations and initiatives in producing countries, to the detriment of the resource and those who will depend on it in the years to come. Perhaps most important is that there is little appreciation for the increasingly critical imbalance between supply and demand.

Can CITES Help?

CITES addresses only a small portion of the medicinal plant issue, but it has the potential to help achieve sustainable and legal trade in medicinal resources. Specifically, CITES can do the following:

- identify trends at the species level and on the global level, to highlight critical issues and address them;
- help to make the trade more transparent, by documenting the species and parts in trade, and volumes traded, because this information is necessary for designing and implementing sustainable management plans;
- stimulate cooperation between importing and exporting countries to ensure that trade is conducted in a legal and sustainable manner;

So What is the Problem?

When the trade is so large, and the implications of unsustainable harvest and trade so serious, why is implementation of CITES for medicinal plants unsatisfactory? Some possible explanations include the following:

- Parties are unaware that CITES-listed medicinal plants are in international trade, because of insufficient knowledge about the parts and derivatives that aretraded.
- Regulatory officials responsible for inspection of plant material are unfamiliar with CITES and do not know that certain traded plant species require CITES documentation.

- Plants are frequently afforded less attention than animal species.
- The variety of parts and derivatives in trade is numerous, and the annotations for CITES- listed medicinal plants vary from species to species, therefore it may be difficult for inspectors to keep track of what should be regulated.
- The majority of trade in medicinal and aromatic plants is not regulated by CITES, and therefore CITES-listed species may be accorded a low priority.

Will these Efforts help Medicinal Plants?

At present the sustainability of the medicinal plant trade is on precarious ground. Through CITES, there is an opportunity to promote sustainable harvest and trade. While regulation is only part of the solution, it is an integral part of a strategy that must entail efforts from many sectors and many directions.

Because of the importance of a sustainable trade in medicinal plants, it is entirely appropriate for CITES to collaborate and indeed advise other global bodies that deal directly with human health issues, on the conservation aspect of this problem. With regard to medicinal plants, the objectives of CITES and the CBD are complementary.

Demand for Medicinal Plants in KwaZulu-Natal

Medicinal plants are used extensively by the black population throughout KwaZulu-Natal (KZN), and indeed South Africa. An active trade and market in medicinal plant material occurs in KwaZulu-Natal as a result of:

- a fragmented distribution of medicinal plant species due to the varied land use, topography and climate in the region,
- large spatial concentrations of consumer demand as more than half the province's population is concentrated in two urban centres,
- local extinctions of plants and the need to access more remote plant populations due to intensive harvesting, and

- various socio-economic factors (including culture and accessible health care) which maintain and stimulate demand.

In KwaZulu-Natal over 400 plants are actively traded [Cunningham 1988; McKean 1996] with an estimated trade volume of some 4 300 tonnes per year. As the market is large and dynamic, several market segments have developed in response to the users' demands and the supply of plants. The extent of trade and the market segments are discussed in the following sections.

Quantity and Trends in Consumer Demand

A survey of several Durban City medical clinics indicated that 53% of the black clinic patients made use of indigenous healers at least once during the previous year, with an average of 3.34 visits in the previous year.

The term indigenous healers or medicine is preferred by the author to the more conventional term traditional healers or medicine. The healing practices used, while originating in African culture, are not purely traditional. The practice is dynamic, addressing new illnesses like AIDS, and adopts new technologies and new medicines.

The healers also deal with all manner of urban social problems, which are not traditional. The term indigenous medicine may therefore be more appropriate as it relates to the practices of healing and divination within an indigenous but modem African culture which may not necessarily be traditional.

While respondents asked whether they visited a indigenous healer in the previous year, the survey omitted to ask respondents whether they purchased indigenous medicine without a healer's prescription. As a consequence, the above estimate of indigenous medicine use may be an underestimate. An indication of the extent of self-medication can be obtained from the expressed preference for hygienically packed medicines.

Eighty-four percent of the black clinic patients indicated that they would prefer more hygienically packed indigenous medicines, indicating that 31% of the sample may not have visited an indigenous healer in 1995 but probably make use of indigenous medicine.

Assuming that the clinic sample is representative of the black population in Durban, the total number of users is estimated to be around 2 million people [that is 84% of 2.442 million blacks resident in Durban (Durban Metropolitan Government 19.96)]. This estimate can be considered a conservative minimum level, as 6% of the indigenous healers patients indicated that they did not make use of western clinics, and therefore using the clinic patients as a proxy for the Durban black population may be a slight underestimate.

The Quantity of Plant Material Reported to be Consumed

Basing the quantity demanded on the reported number of times which the population sample visits indigenous healers (3.34 times per annum), it is estimated that between 900 tonnes and 1 500 tonnes of plant material were consumed in Durban in 1995 .

As most of the estimates are based on relatively imprecise data regarding the numbers of market participants, the broad estimates will generally be rounded off to make for easier reading. However, detailed measurements made within the survey will be retained for descriptive accuracy and where calculations are made.

This estimate assumes that the indigenous medicine users not visiting indigenous healers, that is the remaining 31% of users, would use indigenous medicine at the same rate at which healers are visited (3.34 times a year). The estimate of 900 tonnes is derived if 53% of the population is assumed to use medicine at an average mass of 83.3g per use (the average mass of plant material prescribed by healers and shop traders) and the remaining consumers use the medicine at 216.5g per use (the average mass of plant material traded in the street markets).

The estimate of 1 500 tonnes is obtained if all 84% of the black population uses medicine at 216.5g per use. This last estimate is likely to be more realistic given the extent of wastage associated with the poor storage of plant material.

The Quantity of Plant Material Reported to be Traded

The shop traders are estimated to trade 340 tonnes per year, with approximately 50% reported to be purchased directly from plant gatherers (170 tonnes) and the remaining 50% purchased from street traders (170 tonnes).

The quantities traded by the healers was problematic to estimate due to the unknown number of healers in the survey area. Various reports [Holdstock 1978; Gelfand 1985; Cunningham 1988] had been made regarding the ratio of indigenous healers to the population but these have not been used for a number of reasons.

Firstly, the mode of operation differs considerably between healers, with some healers being extremely busy whilst others may only practise part-time. Secondly, the various healers' organizations have provided a rough indications of the number of healers which are registered with them, but it has not been possible to obtain membership lists from these groups (in addition, the membership makes no differentiation regarding the nature of the practitioners operation, that is, whether it is either full-time or part-time).

Due to the above problems, estimates are based on the visitation frequency reported by the clinic patients and the average number of patients, which the indigenous healers indicate they may treat per day. Following this approach an estimated 936 tonnes of medicinal plants are traded per year by indigenous healers in Durban.

The indigenous healers reported that they purchase plant material from two sources, approximately 50% from the street markets and 50% directly from plant gatherers. This suggests that approximately 468 tonnes are bought from each group.

This estimate uses an average mass of 216.5 g for a prescribed medicine dosage. This mass is the average mass of street traded products and is believed to be a more appropriate mass than the mass dispensed in traders shops and by healers (an average 83.3 g) for estimating the quantity used by healers. The traded products are generally unprocessed and poorly packaged, with a significant proportion (not quantifiable at present) of the plant material spoiled in the transportation and storage process. The author therefore considers the larger street traded mass to be a more accurate reflection of the quantities which healers will utilise but not necessarily dispense.

Of the plant mass traded in the street markets, an estimated 20% of the trade or 220 tonnes, is reported to be traded between the street traders themselves and not to consumers, healers or shop traders. This implies that of the 1 100 tonnes traded in the market as a whole, only 880 tonnes of plant material is the physical stock of plants entering the street markets in a year.

By summing the quantities sold by the various market players to end consumers, it is estimated that some 1 500 tonnes of plant material were sold in the Durban markets in 1996.

This estimate of 1 500 tonnes traded in the market approximates the estimate derived in 4.1.1 regarding the maximum quantity of plant material which may be consumed in Durban given the consumption rates of the clinic patients interviewed. While the two approaches are not entirely independent as both models use a common number in estimating the use associated with healers, there is sufficiently different information in the other sectors which gives confidence to the similarity of estimates.

Potential Provincial and National Consumption Levels

Several studies in different geographic localities throughout South Africa and in different cultural groups have shown that between 58 and 100% of the black population uses indigenous medicine. Holdstock [1978] estimated that between 80 and 85% of the black population in Soweto (a black township in Johannesburg) consumed indigenous medicine. Ellis [1986] found that 100% of a random sample of hospital patients in the Estcourt area (a typical rural population) used indigenous medicine. More recently, a study in peri-urban Bushbuckridge [Mander 1997a] estimated that 58% of the clinic patients used indigenous medicine. However, this estimate is known to be conservative due to the persecution of people suspected of witchcraft in the area, and consequently an unwillingness to admit to the use of indigenous medicine. Assuming that the characteristics of the Durban consumers are representative of the rest of the population in KwaZulu-Natal and South Africa, it is possible to provide a preliminary indication of provincial and national consumption patterns.

In KwaZulu-Natal the current population is estimated to be 8.7 million, with the black population comprising 83% of the total population or 7.2 million people [Central Statistical Services 1996]. Assuming that 84% of the black population use indigenous medicine in KwaZulu-Natal, the number of potential users of indigenous medicine could therefore be 6 million people. Based on an average frequency of uses of 3.34 visits/uses per year (this translates to 20 million uses a year), and assuming an average mass of 216.5g per use, then total quantity of medicinal plants used in KwaZulu-Natal could amount to 4 339 tonnes per year.

Similarly, at a national level there are 33 million blacks in South Africa [Central Statistical Services 1996] with an estimated 28 million (84%) users. Using the same visitation rate per year and the mass per use as above, the total national consumption could amount some 90 million uses per year with a mass of 19 500 tonnes of plant material.

Trends in the Use of Indigenous Medicine

The survey of consumer trends at western clinics and at indigenous healers indicated that a large section of the population has not changed their use patterns, with similar percentages indicating both an increase and a decrease in use. There is, however, an overall increase in the use of indigenous medicine. The following figures (4.3 to 4.8) and discussion outline the changes and reasons for change in use frequency cited by healers and clinic patients.

Of the indigenous healers interviewed, 90% believed that the demand for indigenous medicine would remain high. The shop traders shared the same perspective that trade would remain at high levels.

Discussions with market players and observations of the markets in southern Africa (South Africa, Mozambique, Swaziland, Lesotho and Namibia) have pointed to an increase in the demand for medicines [Scott pers. comm. 1996; Maseko pers. comm. 1997]. While the individual consumers surveyed may not have indicated a trend of increasing use, there is common consensus among traders and researchers that there has been an increase in the number of individuals consuming indigenous medicine. This may be the result of the following factors.

The population growth throughout the region is around 2.4% per year [Central Statistics 1996], leading to an increase in the potential number of people who may make use of indigenous medicine. Coupled with this increase, are the accelerated urbanization rates, which increase the competition for resources and services, especially where economic growth lags behind population growth. Indigenous medicines are actively used to reduce competition for employment, housing, and other social resources that are associated with increasing urban competition. Competition in urban areas may also contribute to psychological stress, and indigenous healing and healers are used extensively to treat stress-related illness.

The existence of poverty also fuels the demand for medicinal plants as households are forced to make use of affordable medicine. While consulting a healer may be more expensive than visiting a clinic, medicines bought directly from the street traders are much cheaper than any other forms of health care, and consequently are an important health care option.

Past government policies in South Africa discriminated against indigenous healing, giving it no positive recognition, and generally labelling the activities as primitive and even legislating against witchcraft practices (Suppression of Witchcraft Act). Perceptions are now changing from several quarters, with increasing official and societal recognition. For example, medical aids in South Africa are increasingly accepting claims, by their members, for visits to indigenous healers [Daily News, 14 January 1997], and black people themselves are developing increasing pride in the culture of indigenous healing.

One of the greatest drivers of the demand for indigenous medicine are the widely held views by the black community that certain illnesses are 'cultural' sicknesses which can only be treated by indigenous medicine. In addition, AIDS is rapidly increasing within the South African community, and with little relief from western medicine, healers report that people with AIDS consult them. There are many healers who now advertise that they have a cure for AIDS, promoting the increased use of indigenous medicine.

Apart from the above, the remote geographical location of many large rural populations also promotes the use of indigenous medicine as it is usually the most accessible source of health care, and the most available health care, as western clinics are either far away or visit rural communities only periodically.

In view of the above factors, the local demand for indigenous medicine is unlikely to decline and will probably increase as the population increases.

Apart from growing local demand, there are also indications of a growing international demand. Neighbouring countries (particularly Namibia and Botswana) are increasing their demand for South African medicinal plants due to the greater diversity, reliability of supply and quantities available. The dry environments have relatively low diversities of high value medicinal plants and in addition, the frequent and regular movement of people between southern African states results in considerable exchange in ideas and information, with foreign healers learning to use South African products. In addition, the declining ability of many countries to maintain the importation of synthetic drugs promotes the continued use of indigenous medicines8. International demand for local plant products is also likely to increase with the growing popularity of alternative medicines and natural products in developed countries [Lange 1997].

For example, discussions in 1996 with women from a remote area in western Mali, reported to the author that they did not bother travelling to the local clinic, in this case only a few kilometres away, as the only medicine which the clinic could provide was quinine and aspirin, and good alternatives for these drugs were more easily accessible in the bush close to where they lived.

Market Segments

Two major market segments, direct consumers and patients of indigenous healers, characterize the market for medicinal plants in KwaZulu-Natal. A third market segment is the pharmaceutical companies, but it is a minor market player at present.

The discussion will focus on the findings for Durban and will make projections for KwaZulu-Natal where appropriate.

Direct Consumers and the Indigenous Healers Patients

This market segment represents those consumers who purchase medicinal products for self-medication from street markets, shops, rural markets, and healers' practices and/or who purchase prescribed medicines from indigenous healers.

The survey was not able to interview direct consumers in the street markets and shops. Nevertheless, observations by the researcher and sales persons in the trade indicated that direct consumers and healers patients came from all socio-economic strata in the black community. Due to the survey limitations and the similarity between the two key market segments, the two market segments will be discussed together with differences indicated where they arise.

The survey was not able to make an assessment of the consumers from street markets and herb shops. The fast nature of transactions and the general pace of activity in the market did not make interviews possible. While sales persons were asked about consumer characteristics, the information obtained was not suitable for detailed analysis as it was based on genera! impressions.

With these limitations, no distinction will be made between the characteristics of the direct consumers (those buying for self-medication) and the healers patients. The report therefore uses the healers' patients as a proxy for the all the indigenous medicine consumers. Some information from the clinic patients is used where appropriate.

The Buyers—Who are They

The majority of users of indigenous African medicine in Durban, and for most of South Africa, are black. They represent a diverse group, with a wide range of social and economic characteristics.

A number of figures are presented to indicate the range of consumer characteristics amongst the indigenous medicine users. At present there is limited use of indigenous medicinal plants by other population groups in South Africa.

This has important implications for the market potential as this study has shown that there is currently little or no differentiation in the products marketed while there are considerable differences in amongst the consumers.

A survey of black clinic patients within Durban indicated that some 53% of the respondents visited indigenous healers in the last year and a further 31% may use indigenous medicine but did not visit healers in the previous year.

Assuming that the clinic sample represents the black population in Durban, then some 1.3 million people may make use of healers every year, with an additional 760 000 people using indigenous medicine without going to a healer, that is, probably purchasing products directly from traders. In total there are approximately 2 million indigenous medicine consumers in Durban, and at a provincial level, basing the estimates on the Durban statistics, there may be some 6 million consumers in KwaZulu-Natal, and 27 million in South Africa.

This assumption is valid as the socio-economic characteristics of the clinic patients are similar to that described by broader studies [Durban Metropolitan Government 1996] of the black population in the Durban region.

This is likely to be a conservative estimate given that some 50% of the population of KwaZulu-Natal is rural, and their frequency of indigenous medicine use is likely to be greater than the urban areas given the limited access to western bio-medical services in remote regions. This is likely to be the case for South Africa as a whole which has similar urban/rural population split.

It is interesting to note that the age-class distribution for the sample tends to mirror the age class distribution for the population as a whole [Durban Metropolitan Government 1996], indicating a broad spectrum of use. One expects that the use of healers would be greater in the older age classes of black society which are more traditional. This is not evident in the study.

The sample used is from the clinic patients as the indigenous healers sample was biased towards females on the days on which the survey was carried out. The survey was undertaken on days when large numbers of patients visited the healers focusing on the treatment of children. Hence the use of the Durban clinic sample as a more representative sample of the user population.

The education category distribution is similar to that recorded for the Durban region [Development Bank of Southern Africa 1994] and indicates that the sample selected is a relatively accurate representation of the Durban population. Past speculation has predicted that low education levels would be strongly correlated to the use of indigenous medicine. However, that over 60% of the consumers have at least some form of secondary education. Higher education levels do not appear to result in a reduction in the consumption of indigenous medicine.

One may also expect that certain religious affiliations are likely to influence the use of indigenous medicine, given the magic and ancestral worship associated with its use. The survey indicates that 96% of the consumers had a Christian affiliation.

A broad spectrum of occupational classes are represented in the survey sample. What is clear that the use of indigenous medicine is not confined to the lower earning occupations. This is confirmed in the figure illustrating the wide range of incomes earned by the consumers' household.

Confirms the wide range of the people that make use of indigenous medicine. The range includes, people from conservative traditional backgrounds (the traditional homesteads), relatively wealthy people (big houses), average people (4-roomed house), recent migrants to the city, new families, and people affected by political violence (the shacks), and single people and poor people (the hostels and rented rooms). The diversity in the types of homes which consumers live in provides an indication of the diversity of social and economic backgrounds of the users.

The above discussion shows that the majority of the black population in Durban is making use of indigenous medicine irrespective of religion, age, education and economic status. The direct consumers and the healers patients represent a large consumer population with considerable socio-economic diversity within the group. This has important implications for the market's development.

The Products Purchased

The products consumed are generally unrefined plant medicines with limited processing apart from grinding, chopping, and mixing. Raw plant material is frequently bought directly by consumers who may grind it themselves following instructions provided by the healers or traders. Plant products are taken as medicines in the following forms:

- infusions (chopped bark, leaves, seeds/fruit, stems, bulbs, rhizomes and roots steeped in water) which can be drunk, used as an emetic, or as an enema,
- concentrates (infusions where the water is boiled off concentrating the liquid) which are usually drunk,
- inhalants (plant parts or powdered parts burnt to produce smoke or boiled to produce steam) which is breathed in,
- powder (ground plant parts, usually tree bark, roots and leaves - usually burnt or raw) and which can be licked, used as snuff, bathed with, rubbed on to the skin, or implanted under the skin,
- poultices (fresh leaves of fleshy plants) applied to wounds, sores, and other skin ailments, and
- protective charms (live or dried plants) used for planting or scattering around the homestead.

The Quantities Demanded

The Durban survey estimated that some 1 500 tonnes of plant material was consumed per annum. The average mass per plant product bought in the street markets was 216.5g, and was 83g per product in the traders' shops. Observations in the street markets indicated that customers usually purchased one item in the street market, whereas in the traders' shops, customers tended to buy more than one product.

The shop traders reported that the customers buy on average 127.2g per visit or 1.5 items per visit. At the healers' practices, the customers purchased similar quantities to those traded by the shop traders but it was usually only one item per visit.

The healers' patients did not select the quantity purchased but were prescribed a quantity by the dispensing healer. In addition, the item purchased was usually a mixture of various plant species (which is generally confidential information).

The indigenous healers' patients or customers consumed some 61% of the market produce (936 tonnes), while the direct consumers bought 22% of the market produce from traders' shops (340 tonnes) and 17% from street traders (256 tonnes).

Patients refers to someone who is prescribed a medicine, whereas a customer is someone who purchases a product from the healer's stock without a consultation.

At a provincial level, the consumers demand approximately 4339 tonnes a year and nationally some 19 500 tonnes may be consumed.

The Timing of Purchases

Consumers visited indigenous healers on average 3.34 times a year and visited the markets towards end of the month when salaries were paid. Purchases of medicine were generally associated with doing other regular chores, such as travelling to work or going shopping. Visiting indigenous healers on the other hand usually involved a specific journey to the healer but with other activities attached.

This estimate is used to predict the visitation frequency of the entire user population (healers' patients and direct consumers) as the survey did not collect information on the frequency of indigenous medicine use (as opposed to the frequency of visiting a healer).

Observations of the market, and interviews indicated that there was greater buying activity on Mondays, Fridays and particularly Saturdays. Limited purchasing took place on Sundays. The time of purchases from shops and the street was normally between 10h00 and 16h00 during weekdays and on Saturdays between 10h00 and 14h00. Patients visiting healers tended to follow similar weekly patterns, but started earlier in the day. Patients arrived at the healers' practices between 07h30 until about 16h00 during weekdays, and up to 13h00 on Saturdays.

Consumption of certain species was generally constant throughout the year with a small peak in demand for chest-related medicines during the winter months and a small peak for homestead blessing products at the end of the year. The climate in Durban is tropical and consequently has a limited winter peak for chest-related medicines. In contrast, healers and traders in colder regions have reported substantial increases in the demand for Siphonochilus, Alepidea and Warburgia during the winter months (June, July and August in southern Africa).

The Reasons for Purchasing Indigenous Medicine

Consumers buy medicinal plants for a range of reasons as discussed. Various experts and authorities have speculated that the high demand for indigenous medicine by the black population in South Africa is due to low income, poor education opportunities, high costs of western medicine, and the lack of clinics.

An analysis of clearly the perspective that access to clinics and the cost of western medicines were not important considerations in determining the use of healers. On the other hand, strong sentiments were expressed regarding the desire for using indigenous health care systems and there was also strong support for the notion that clinics could not cure particular ailments. Respondents made it quite clear that the selection of healing systems depended on the type of illnesses or problems that they were experiencing. This indicates that in many cases, there are not western alternatives to the services provided by indigenous medicine. The survey obtained clear evidence indicating that black people in Durban make use of both the western and indigenous health care systems.

The survey showed little or no evidence of any positive relationship between low education and income levels and a higher frequency of visits to healers. On the contrary, the healers' customers reported that they would continue to use indigenous medicine even if it became more expensive. In view of the above attitudes, indigenous medicine could be classified as a basic consumer good, such food, clothing, western medicine and housing.

In fact, consumers reported that indigenous healers were already more expensive than western medicine.

While the cost of consulting healers may be relatively expensive when compared to clinics, it is important to note that self-medication, using indigenous medicines, was the cheapest form of health care available.

This is especially relevant to rural communities. Unlike the cities, where clinics may be relatively easily accessible, rural areas have few clinics and consequently rural communities have little or no choice in the health care systems used. Indigenous health care being the only accessible system for a large proportion of the people given the distances to travel to clinics and the costs of transport.

The Purchasing Power of Consumers

The purchasing power of consumers can be considered from the perspective of the household or from the individual consumer. Household income is discussed above and shows that there is a wide range in purchasing power, with the majority earning relatively low incomes and therefore individuals having limited purchasing power. However, purchasing power is unlikely to be a significant limitation when buying products for self-medication as this could amount to US$ 1.50 (R 6.70) (the cost of two beers) per year for an individual consumer or US$ 9 (R 40) per household per year.

Using an average of 3.34 purchases of indigenous medicine per year.

The average household size for healers' customers is six people.

On the other hand, consulting an indigenous healer is likely to represent a significant cost as the average consulting fee (US$ 8.2 or R37) and associated prescribed medicine is some 18 times more expensive than the average cost of medicine bought at the markets for self-medication, and could cost an individual consumer around US$ 28 (R 124) per year. The costs to a household (of six people) could amount to US$ 168 (R 744) per year. The average monthly income earned by households visiting healers is between US$ 178 (R 800) to US$ 333 (R 1 500) per month. Consequently, the average household could spend between one half a month's income (4.2% of annual income) and one month's income (8.3% of annual income) on indigenous medicine per year.

The traders (street, shops and healers) indicated that at least 75% of their customers accepted the price charged, with the remainder bargaining for a lower price. This may indicate that for most consumers, the prices charged are affordable.

While the purchasing power of a large segment of the population is limited due to low income and relatively high costs (in prescribed medicine), it is unlikely to be limited for purchasing products for self-medication. In addition, the consumers indicated that their demand would remain the same irrespective of high prices.

'High prices' are probably relative to past experiences of price increases which, if considered by percentage, are considerable (for example, 50% increases in prices are common). However, given the real amount of money involved (US$ 0.11 or R 0.50 increase per product purchased) and the infrequent use of indigenous medicine, it does not constitute a significant cost.

At a community level, the purchasing power of the user group in Durban is significant and amounts to some US$ 1.02 billion (R 4.6 billion) per year. The survey has shown that the demand for indigenous medicine is relatively inelastic, that is, the consumers consider indigenous medicine as a basic consumer good which needs to be purchased to maintain their well-being. Consequently, there is a high degree of certainty that considerable sums of money will be spent on indigenous medicine on an annual basis in Durban. Using the estimated annual expenditure per household on indigenous medicine (between 4.2% and 8.3% of annual household income), then one can estimate that between US$ 42 million (R 190 million) and US$ 84 million (R 380 million) could be spent per annum in Durban.

This estimate is based on a user population of 2 million, with an average monthly income of R1 150 (US$ 256) and an average household size of six people [Development Bank of Southern Africa, 1994].

Using the quantities of plants traded and the average price of raw products bought (R 14/kg), it is possible to estimate the value of expenditure on raw plant products.

These values are the trade in raw products and exclude any value-added through processing or prescription.

In Durban some 1 500 tonnes were traded and this would have generated an expenditure of US$ 4.7 million (R 21 million) per annum.

In KwaZulu-Natal, the trade of 4 300 tonnes would have generated an expenditure of some US$ 13.3 million (R 60 million) per annum. This is approximately one-third of the value of the annual maize harvest in KwaZulu-Natal.

At a national level, a trade of 19 500 tonnes would generate an expenditure of US$ 61 million (R 273 million) per annum (assuming the average price of Durban products).

Who are the Buyers: Several pharmaceutical companies are currently developing products for the African market in South Africa. There are reports that some companies are buying raw materials from plant harvesters in rural areas. One pharmaceutical company, which has a major share of the domestic market for western bio-medical products, is currently establishing partnerships to cultivate plants for their production process. Very little information is available regarding the pharmaceutical companies given the high degree of competition and secrecy that exists.

It is known that one of the companies is currently focusing on producing products for the upper-end of the consumer market. The large pharmaceutical company, is also focusing on products which would be registered by the Medicines Control Council, which has high standards matching the conventions in Europe and North America.

Quantities Demanded: The quantity of plants demanded is unknown at present, and is likely to remain so for the short term until the practices become more established and transparent.

The Products Purchased: A small number of plants are being focused on due to the high costs of pharmacological screening and testing. Some 10 to 20 species are probably the focus of current formal commercial activities. The focus is also likely to be on species, which are relatively easily cultivated to ensure that commercial production can be sustained.

Commercial activities undertaken by conventional businesses (in the western sense) rather than informal markets which dominate the current trade in indigenous medicine.

The Timing of Purchases: Whilst the products are still being developed and consumer preferences have not been tested in the market place, the timing of purchases is likely to be unknown.

The Reasons for Purchases: Pharmaceutical companies purchase material to process and trade to consumer outlets. The business opportunities associated with the large numbers of indigenous medicine consumers have, until recently, been largely ignored by the pharmaceutical industry. Recent research into the size of the indigenous medicine market has fuelled considerable interest by local companies.

The Purchasing Power: The purchasing power of large pharmaceutical industries is considerable relative to other market players in the trade. The access of large corporations to finance is far greater than the monies available to the operators in the current indigenous medicine trade. However, despite the greater purchasing power, established pharmaceutical companies are unlikely to purchase large volumes of material from existing traders, due to the unreliability of supply and current legislation.

The Supply of Medicinal Plants in KwaZulu-Natal

This study has established that the large volume of indigenous medicinal plants, which is traded in the southern African markets, is harvested from wild populations, with insignificant cultivation taking place. These plants are harvested from within South Africa and from neighbouring countries such as Swaziland, Lesotho, Mozambique and Namibia. The supply of high value plants has declined leading to concerns within the industry and conservation agencies.

Sources of Supply

Medicinal plants supplied to the markets in KwaZulu-Natal are harvested from a wide range of habitats in the region, including coastal forests, coastal grasslands, mangroves, swamp forests, grasslands, woodlands, riverine forest, montane forest, wetlands, and sub-alpine grasslands. These habitats are located on communal lands, commercial farms, forestry estates, protected areas, and in neighbouring countries.

Domestic Sources: The majority of the plants are harvested from wild populations on communal lands. Popular species, which are no longer available in these communal areas, may be harvested on forestry estates (exotic plantations with natural areas), commercial farms, and protected areas. Harvesting takes place with or without the consent of the landowners or local authority. There is limited commercial cultivation of medicinal species for local markets, although several organizations, such as Silverglen Medicinal Nursery, Institute of Natural Resources, Mondi Forests (a timber company) and several conservation agencies are promoting the cultivation of medicinal plants by farmers and other commercial enterprises.

Supply from wild populations in communal areas: The main source of plants for markets in KwaZulu-Natal is from communal or tribal lands where there is generally easy access to forest and grassland resources. In South Africa, there has been an erosion of tribal authority, and little or no state support for developing management systems for communal natural resources. Consequently, there are limited skills and motivation to promote natural resource management in these areas. This has led to a situation where rural communities take little or no responsibility for the state of their natural resources, allowing individuals in the community or outsiders to exploit medicinal plant populations with little or no control [Mander 1997a].

The communal areas closest to the urban and rural markets have been the primary focus of harvesting activities. However, as high value or popular plants have been depleted in these areas, harvesting of popular and scarce species takes place in more and more distant areas.

The location of the main harvesting areas has increased in distance from Durban, with an average increase in travel time6 of 45% (or 2 hours) over 8 years, between the source and market. The change in travel time ranges between an increase of 1 hour to 4 hours. For example, Eucomis autumnalis, a formerly common grassland bulb which was harvested largely within two hours travel, is now being extensively harvested in areas of 4 to 5 hours away. Furthermore, other barriers to trade, such as international borders and the associated trade controls, are increasingly being encountered and overcome in order to meet the demand for plants. Six out of the nine most popular medicinal species being studied (66%) are now being harvested in either Swaziland and/or Mozambique, and transported to the Durban markets for sale.

Travel time has been used to give an indication of changes in the distance between the markets and the source as it represents a more realistic barrier in the market than distance.

The declining size of bulbs and thickness of bark also illustrate the scarcity of plants. Indigenous healers have reported that they are increasingly using smaller sizes of plants, indicating that popular plants are getting less and less opportunity to grow and to reproduce. Between 25% and 39% of the healers indicated that, for the nine popular plants, they were now using smaller sizes than before. Between 8% and 15% of the healers indicated that they were now using different plant parts.

The general lack of willingness and/or ability to enforce property rights associated with plants in the region, combined with the high levels of poverty in rural areas, exacerbates the destructive methods of harvesting. Rural women are desperate to generate a cash income, and will therefore harvest large numbers of plants for sale to the markets. Sustainable harvesting is not practised, as harvesters have no guarantees that they will benefit from any wise harvesting of species. The above factors result in a highly destructive approach to harvesting with each high value plant population becoming depleted, leading to a new focus on either a different species or on a further area which may still have high value plants.

A further destructive condition, which impacts on plant populations, is the fact that most women harvesters concentrate their activities in one area. They are unlikely to shift to new areas to look for a particular species due to travel costs, and will focus on different species to harvest. This means that a population of popular species will not be given a chance to regenerate as any individual popular plant seen while in the course of gathering other plants, will be collected. Consequently, popular species face localized extinctions in areas where harvesters regularly gather medicinal plants for the market.

As consequence of the above approaches to harvesting, the supply of indigenous plants from communal areas is declining, leading to a shortage of popular plants in the market. The local extinctions and concomitant increasing distance to harvesting locations, and the declining size of the plants utilized by healers, are clear indicators that the current supply of plants from communal areas is not sustainable. This has resulted in an increase in imports and an increasing interest in cultivation.

Supply from Commercial Farms: There are several commercial operations initiating the cultivation of indigenous plants to supply markets. Production is focused on supplying high value plants to pharmaceutical companies either within South Africa or in European markets. Production for the South African market is believed to be limited to a few species that can be registered with the Medicines Control Council. In

KwaZulu-Natal there are low supplies of plants from commercial farms.

Due to the infancy of large-scale commercial ventures in the indigenous medicine markets and the lack products on the market, there is considerable secrecy in the industry. Little information will be available until products are openly traded.

The level of harvesting from undeveloped areas on commercial farms is unknown. The localities identified by the plant gatherers indicate that there is limited harvesting on commercial land. There is however, some illegal harvesting from commercial farms or estates. There has been an increasing awareness amongst landowners regarding the value of medicinal plants, and it is unlikely that any large-scale harvesting takes place on commercial farms. Harvesting plants for home consumption by farm labourers is likely to be the largest form of use on these properties.

Imports: A number of plant species are imported into South Africa (including KwaZulu-Natal) for the medicinal plant trade. The imports take place on an informal basis with no documentation or customs authorization. There is considerable labour migration between Lesotho, Swaziland, Mozambique and South Africa, and this promotes a large informal movement of plant material. Rural families from neighbouring countries frequently have members of their households or community working within South Africa, particularly in large cities, thereby providing remote locations with market information and transport mechanisms. The material is usually traded in its raw form and can be either sold on street markets, in shops, by healers or by wholesalers.

Popular species, now becoming increasingly difficult to obtain in South Africa, are the main focus of trade. Discussions in the Durban market have indicated that Haworthia limifolia, Boweia volubilis and Warburgia salutaris are imported in large quantities from Swaziland and Mozambique. These two countries are now recognized as the main sources of supply for these species. Two other species in great demand, Alepidea amatymbica and Eucomis autumnalis, are imported from Lesotho but in small quantities.

The different sources of imports can be ascribed to the distribution of species. All of these species are still found in South Africa but the declining local supply and increasing inaccessibility has led to the importation of these species from countries where they are still common and/or easily accessible.

The quantities of plants imported into South Africa are unknown. The informal nature of the plant trade and the illegal nature of imports make it difficult to make any quantitative estimates of the quantities imported into South Africa. For one species, Warburgia salutaris, it may be possible to provide some idea of what is being imported due to the localized extinction that has occurred in parts of South Africa. The market survey estimated that some 17 tonnes of Warburgia salutaris were traded in Durban in 1996 and Williams pers. comm. 1997 suggests that between 10 and 20 tonnes were traded in Gauteng (formerly the Johannesberg area) in 1995.

As the Durban and Gauteng markets are the major trading conduits, it is likely that between 30 to 40 tonnes of Warburgia salutaris are imported annually from Mozambique and Swaziland. Some of the other species, such as Boweia volubilis, Siphonochilus aethiopicus, Curtisia dentata, Eucomis autumnalis, and Haworthia limifolia are also imported to some degree but the quantities are unknown. For example, 33% of the traders selling Boweia volubilis (or nine traders), indicated that they obtained their plants in Mozambique.

Current and Potential Production

The current production of plant material for the market is unknown but can be based on the estimates made in Section regarding consumer demand. The total quantity of plant material supplied to the markets in Durban is 1 500 tonnes a year, and for KwaZulu (including Durban) it is estimated to be some 4 300 tonnes a year. At national level it is suggested that some 19 500 tonnes may be traded. However, these quantities should not be considered as production but rather as harvesting since little or no cultivation or processing takes place.

The above quantities are harvested from wild populations and consequently the stock of plants is not known. It is thus not possible with our present level of knowledge to predict the potential production of these wild stocks. However, what is known, is that for many species the current levels of harvesting are not sustainable. Observations of the market indicate that a number of species are becoming scarce, with concomitant price increases, increasing imports, irregular supply, reductions in the size and/or thickness of plant products, and increasing use of substitute plants. For example:

- Siphonochilus aethiopicus - sells for between 10 and 30 times the average price of other popular plants in the market.
- Ocotea bullata - alternative tree species (Cryptocarya spp.) in the Laurel family is increasingly being used as a substitute.
- Warburgia salutaris - sells for double the average price of other bark products and is mostly imported from Mozambique.
- Eucomis autumnalis - the average size of bulbs is getting smaller and they are frequently unobtainable in the markets.
- Alepidea amatymbica - previously a common species in the province is now being imported from the Eastern Cape and Lesotho, or being collected in more distant localities. Its price is increasing and market players are finding it increasingly difficult to maintain their preferred stock levels.
- Boweia volubilis - large bulbs are scarce and sell for more than three times the price (per unit weight) of small bulbs.

Prices refer to price per kilogram and not to price per unit.

The above examples describe the market conditions for some of the most popular medicinal plants traded, showing the effects of trade on species. This evidence is supported by the observations of market players. For the nine popular species, between 45% and 55% of the healers reported that the sale of plants had increased (largely due to increasing demand). However, for these same species, between 19% and 30% of the healers indicated that sales had declined due to scarcity. Healers who are less well connected or who have fewer financial/ transport resources are likely to have less access to any species that may become scarce.

Sixty percent of the healers interviewed indicated that they used substitute plants, showing the degree to which shortages may occur in the market.

The harvesting technique used in gathering plant material is highly destructive contributing to the decline in supply to markets. Of the most important plants traded in the markets, approximately 28% of the plants have the whole plant or bulb harvested. A further 63% of the plants have either their roots or bark harvested, which for small plants would imply that the whole plant would be extracted from the ground, and for large plants it would imply a high risk of death due to damage to the plant. For scarce species, ring-barking is frequently practised to maximize the harvest of bark, usually causing the death of the tree.

The scale of harvesting, the destructive methods used, and the lack of cultivation have contributed to a widespread decline in plant populations throughout the province and surrounding areas. This has led to considerable concern regarding the sustainability of supply. For example, studies by Cunningham [1988] indicate that harvesting levels, at the time of his work, were not sustainable.

In southern Natal forests, some 51% of Ocotea bullata trees and 57% of Curtisia dentata trees were estimated to have more than 50% of their bark removed. In Maputaland, all Warburgia salutaris trees greater than 5 cm in diameter (at breast height), located in the study (excluding protected areas), had been debarked. Similarly, for an area closer to Durban, Oatley [1979] estimated that 99% of some 450 Ocotea bullata located, had their bark damaged and Cooper [1979] estimated that for six areas where he had been working, some 95% of the Ocotea bullata had been damaged, with 45% of the trees ring-barked and dying.

There has been some cultivation of popular medicinal species by Silverglen Medicinal Nursery, Natal Parks Board, the

Institute of Natural Resources, and Mondi Forests. This production is however not intended for markets but rather for research, education, and to provide foundation stocks for further propagation. These activities therefore do not provide a significant source of supply. There is also a growing number of healers beginning to cultivate plants for their own practices but these are as yet insignificant in terms of the volumes produced. There is one farmer in KwaZulu-Natal currently cultivating Siphonochilus aethiopicus for the indigenous medicinal trade within KwaZulu-Natal.

Potential Production of Market Materials

The decline in access to plant species indicates that current harvesting levels are not sustainable, and it can be anticipated that unless management and/or propagation is undertaken greater shortages of plant material are likely to occur in the future.

The supply of other popular species can also be expected to decline in the future. It is possible that currently popular species may face local extinctions, as has already happened for Warburgia salutaris and Siphonochilus aethiopicus.

Current market trends have indicated that plant populations will continue to decline in the future while harvesting is not managed and demand is sustained. The areas for potential harvesting have been reduced significantly, with the area of grasslands, savannah and thicket being reduced from 72 000 km^2 to 29 000 km^2. A 60% reduction in harvestable grasslands and savannah area has taken place due to land use changes and past harvesting pressure.

The reduction in area does not imply that all medicinal species have been removed from the area, but rather that the popular and high value species are present in minimal quantities.

The potential area of forests which are available for harvesting have been reduced from 889 km^2 to 260 km^2. A 70% reduction in harvestable area has occurred through the intensive use of forests not protected by either conservation agencies or private land owners.

Grassland, Savannah and Thicket Biomes—the Area Available for Plant Harvesting

Grassland, savannah and thicket biome	*Area*
Total area in KwaZulu-Natal[1]	85415 km^2
Total area protected[1]	7687 km^2 (9%)
Area not protected and undeveloped[2]	72000 km^2
Land area already developed (timber and crops)[2]	17000 km^2
Potential area available for harvesting	55000 km^2
Available area (communal lands) already intensively harvested[2]	26000 km^2
Area available for future harvesting with limited past commercial harvesting (commercial farm)	29000 km^2

[1] Low and Robelo 1996

[2] Department of Agriculture 1997

Forest Biomes—the Area Available for Plant Harvesting

Forest biome (sand, coastal and Afro-montane)	*Areas*
Total area in KwaZulu-Natal[1]	1185 km^2
Total area protected[1]	298 km^2 (25%)
Potential area available for harvesting	889 km^2
Forest area on commercial farms with limited past commercial harvesting[2]	260 km^2
Area (generally communal lands) already intensively harvested	629 km^2

For both groups of biomes, the protected areas, plantations, crop-lands, and developed land have been excluded. These areas could not be utilized due to either the absence of indigenous plants or the protective legislation governing the use of indigenous plants.

The previous discussions on supply indicate that common property areas in KwaZulu-Natal have largely been exhausted of the high value and popular species, with the only areas of high potential remaining on private property or in more distant locations out of the province. There has however been selected exploitation of scarce forest species (Ocotea bullata) on private properties in KwaZulu-Natal [Cooper 1985], indicating that the estimates made for available forest resources may be too high.

The greater reduction in forest area compared to grasslands/savannah, can be ascribed to equal popularity of grassland/savannah and forest species. Of the 68 species identified by street traders and plant gatherers as being important trade items, 49% were forest species and 51% were grassland and savannah species.

The intensity of harvesting in forests has therefore been considerably higher than harvesting in grasslands and savannah, with the area of forests being some 61 times smaller than the available area of grasslands/savannah. The grassland and savannah species used tend to be dominated by plant forms with short life cycles such as bulbs and rhizomes, while forest species used are dominated by bark producing trees, which take many years to mature.

Assuming that the proportions of plant species used from the respective vegetation biomes was matched by the mass of plants used (that is, 51% of the species represented 51% of the mass traded), then the forests would need to produce some 8.1 tonnes per km^2 per annum, while the grasslands would need to produce some 78 kg per km^2 per annum. These are not accurate estimates, but are rather an illustration of the orders of magnitude of supply constraints and opportunities within the different biomes.

Method used to estimate production required from remaining underutilised vegetation biomes: Grassland and savanna biome: (51% x 4 300 tonnes of marketed materials in KwaZulu-Natal) = (2 193 tonnes)/28 000 km^2 of available grasslands and savanna = 78 kg per km^2 Forest biome: (49% x 4 300 tonnes of marketed materials in KwaZulu-Natal) = (2 107 tonnes)/260 km2 =8 100 kg per km^2.

The above discussion regarding potential areas for harvesting indicates that grasslands and savannahs on commercial farms could be managed on a sustainable basis to supply material for the plant markets. A large grassland and savannah area remains relatively underutilized in terms of medicinal plant harvesting. However, forests on commercial farms would be unlikely to be able to supply sufficiently large quantities of medicinal plants for the market in KwaZulu-Natal.

The sustained harvesting of 78 kg a km^2 per annum may be feasible in grasslands and savannah, while the harvesting of 8.1 tonnes per km^2 per annum of material from existing forests would not be sustainable. The implications of the above are that grassland species could be managed to supply plants for the market in the short term, while forests could only produce the required volumes in the long term provided extensive enrichment planting and management takes place.

Another option to sustain and possibly increase supply is cultivation. Experience in South Africa has indicated that it is possible to cultivate medicinal species in farming systems. The economic feasibility is however unknown. Experiences in India, China and USA have shown that it is possible to produce large volumes of medicinal plants for the market [Lambert et al. 1996]. This implies that it would be possible to produce sufficient plant volumes to meet the demand for indigenous medicinal plants in South Africa should the necessary levels of farm investment take place. However, while it may be possible to supply large quantities of bulbs, tubers, and herbs in the short term, it would take considerably longer to produce sufficient bark products to meet market demand. The slow growing nature of several popular tree species implies that should large-scale production take place, it is unlikely that an increase in the production of bark products would be feasible in the short to medium term.

There is one option that could be used as an interim measure to enhance the supply of several popular tree species in the short term. Medicinal tree species, such as Ocotea bullata and Curtisia dentata, are harvested as high value timber from southern Cape indigenous forests. This harvesting provides a potential bi-product in the form of bark for the medicinal plant trade. The quantities produced in the southern Cape would need to be investigated.

Quantities by Products

The market survey focused on the market as a whole as well as on nine popular species.

Mass Traded Within the Market

Trading area	*Quantities traded per annum*
Durban City (including surrounding areas)	1519 tonnes
KwaZulu-Natal (province)	4339 tonnes
South Africa	19500 tonnes

The total tonnage traded in Durban has been estimated to be some 1 500 tonnes per year. The products included would consist of bulbs (making up a large proportion of the mass), bark, tubers and herbs. The Durban estimates can be used to provide an indication of regional and national quantities assuming the similarities in the population.

The survey also collected detailed information on nine popular species in Durban and the annual mass of these plants traded are illustrated in descending order.

Quantities of Nine Popular Species Sold in the Durban Medicinal Trade

Botanical Name	*Zulu Name*	*Tonnes traded per year*
Scilla natalensis	Inguduza	95.5
Eucomis autumnalis	Umathunga	73.2
Boweia volubilis	Igibisila	43
Alepidea amatymbica	Ikhathazo	31.2
Ocotea bullata	Unukani	25.3
Curtisia dentata	Umlahleni	23.9
Haworthia limifolia1	Umathithibala	22.5
Warburgia salutaris	Isibhaha	17.2
Siphonochilus aethiopicus1	Indungulo	1.9

Scilla natalensis is a popular bulb with little supply constraints yet and with large populations still extant within the province. This serves to provide a context for understanding the levels of trade in other popular species. Bulbous species can be expected to contribute to greater proportions of the trade (on a weight basis) given the high moisture content within bulbs, hence the top three masses are all bulb species. However, what is useful to note is that the volume of Boweia traded is approximately half that of Scilla natalensis, probably a result of both greater scarcity and less demand. In terms of the bark traded, it can be seen that 30% less Warburgia salutaris is traded relative to the two other popular barks, even though it is considered to be one of the most popular medicines.

This can be ascribed to the scarcity of the plant within South Africa. Siphonochilus aethiopicus is traded in low volumes due to the scarcity of the plants and the relatively small mass of the products sold. The total mass of the nine popular species (2% of species traded) amounts to approximately 22% of the total tonnage traded in Durban every year.

The numbers of plants/units traded for the nine most popular species have been estimated and are listed. While there were considerable differences between species in the overall mass sold, it is interesting to note that in terms of the bulbs and succulents, the range in numbers sold was similar, that is, between 310 000 and 480 000 plants were used per year. For the trees, the range is between 1 400 and 2 100 trees used per year. Alepidea amatymbica rates as the highest number sold as, on average, four plants are sold in every transaction.

In terms of mass, the greatest quantity traded (Scilla natalensis) is some 51 times greater than the lowest quantity traded (Siphonochilus aethiopicus), while in terms of numbers, the greatest number sold (Alepidea amatymbica) is some 35 times more that the least numbers sold (again Siphonochilus aethiopicus).

Number of Plants and the Units Traded for the Nine most Popular Species

Botanical name	*Number of purchases made per year*[1]	*Equivalent plants used per year*[2]	*Plant material used*
Curtisia dentata	548000	1494	Tree bark
Ocotea bullata	529000	1581	Tree bark
Warburgia salutaris	514000	1075	Tree bark

Contd...

Botanical name	*Number of purchases made per year*[1]	*Equivalent plants used per year*[2]	*Plant material used*
Haworthia limifolia	479000	479000	Whole plant
Alepidea amatymbica	455000	1820000	Herb root
Scilla natalensis	432000	432000	Bulb
Eucomis autumnalis	428000	428000	Bulb
Boweia volubilis	386000	386000	Bulb
Siphonochilus aethiopicus[3]	67142	52800	Rhizome

[1] The number of purchases is based on the mean mass of plant material purchased per sale (either a part of a plant, a whole plant or many plants) at the time of the survey.

[2] The equivalent plant numbers are based on the total annual market mass traded divided by; in the case of a bulb, root, rhizome or whole plant, the mean market mass per entire plant, and in the case of trees, by an assumed mass of 16 kg (dry weight) of harvested bark per tree. This assumption is based on average mass derived from bark harvested from three of the most popular bark species traded.

[3] Siphonochilus aethiopicus is frequently sold in shops and healers' practices in pieces (at a mean mass of 6 g) due to high prices, while in the street markets it is usually sold whole (at a mean mass of 35.6 g). An average sale mass of 21 g is used to estimate the number of sales, while the average mass of whole plants is used to estimate the numbers of plants sold.

Description of Producers

The current producers of material for the Durban markets are rural women, who harvest a wide range of plant material from mainly communal lands. There are no costs incurred in the cultivation of plants as only wild populations are harvested, although there are harvesting and transport costs. Women gathering plants for trade to the market came from a wide range of geographical locations. Of the 55 different areas identified as home locations, 24% lived within 100 km from Durban; 33% lived between 100 km to 200 km away from Durban; and 45% lived between 200 km to 500+ km away from Durban. The largest number of gatherers originated from distant localities in communal areas.

The general harvesting approach used is for individuals or groups of women to scout around in the various vegetation associations within their immediate vicinity. Gatherers interviewed indicated that they may be assisted by, on average, one (Ezimbuzini market) and 1.6 (Russel Street market) other people in harvesting activities. Any plants considered marketable, based on observations of the markets and/or from reports from associates, are collected. Marketability depends on both the species, the size of the plant and the time of month/year. Gatherers tend to concentrate their harvesting during the month and then market their products towards the end of the month. This harvesting approach results in a peak in marketing around the end of the month. The end of the year also produces a peak in trade, especially for live plants.

A range of basic implements is used to harvest material. Bark is harvested by using an axe or cane knife (machete). Bulbs and roots are dug up using a hoe, metal rod or similar metal instrument. During the winter months there are relatively fewer bulbs harvested due to the aerial plant parts dying back and the plants becoming less visible. The advent of summer and the development of leaves and flower heads, results in a reversal of this trend.

The plants are placed in woven plastic sacks and generally carried on their heads back to the homestead. Harvests are accumulated until quantities are large enough to warrant a journey to the market. Bark products are usually dried before being transported to the market. Little other processing takes place.

Many of the gatherers in KwaZulu-Natal travel to the Durban markets themselves, and there they can undertake some processing, depending on the species traded and the experience of the gatherers. The unprocessed products consisted of whole live plants such as Haworthia, Clivia, Gasteria, and numerous bulb species. Partially processed products consisted of sections or chunks of plant parts such as roots, tubers, branches, bark, and bulbs. Products with greater levels of processing consisted of unmixed chopped and ground bark. The most sophisticated processed products were special mixtures, such as 'ntelezi' and 'ubulawu', consisting of mixtures of chopped bark and bulbs and other plant parts.

In Durban it is estimated that there are approximately 7,500 gatherers selling material directly to healers. Healers reported that they have on average five gatherers collecting for their practices. In addition, some 670 gatherers traded their produce in the street markets. In total, over 8,000 gatherers harvest materials for the Durban market. Similarly, using Durban as a proxy for KwaZulu-Natal, it is estimated that there would be at least another 8 000 gatherers given that approximately half the population of KwaZulu-Natal resides in and around Durban [Development Bank of Southern Africa 1994].

The incomes earned by the rural gatherers are a very important household resource. In the Russel Street and Ezimbizini Street markets, the gatherers earned an average of US$ 98 (R 440) and US$ 67 (R 300) per month, respectively. While these amounts are only 56% and 38% of the minimum wage in South Africa (Wage Act, Act 5 of 1957), it nevertheless represents a significant income, as in most cases there are few alternative income sources in underdeveloped rural areas. The cash incomes are important, providing rural women with monies for consumer goods.

While individual gatherers are the major producers for the market there are two other groups which also harvest products for the market. There are entrepreneurs, which may hire casual labour to harvest bulk quantities of plants. Their general modus operandi is to transport gatherers into localities, which are known to have abundant supplies of valuable plants. Harvesting takes place, and the products are then transported back to the entrepreneurs' shop or practice. The other group of producers are the indigenous healers themselves. Many Durban healers reported that they would on occasion collect plant material themselves. This takes place in special cases when specific rituals have to be performed in the harvesting of the plants. However, the Durban healers reported that they would only do this once or twice a year. In rural areas, the healers are more active in collecting plants.

As mentioned in Section 5.2, there is a movement amongst healers to start growing medicinal plants for their own practices. While this activity is limited at present, the demand for assistance and plant resources is growing in both rural and urban areas. The information and learning opportunities provided by various organizations regarding the propagation potential of medicinal plants is leading to increasing numbers of healers starting to produce plants at their homesteads. The numbers involved are however unknown at present but appear relatively insignificant given the total quantity of plants used in the industry.

The present focus of production (or more aptly termed harvesting) are the communal areas. There is however active but illegal harvesting within protected areas, private commercial farms and forestry estates. During the course of research, several gatherers have indicated that they have intimate knowledge of selected plant populations within protected or private areas. These areas are likely to play an increasingly important role in production as the population of high value species declines in more accessible areas.

Competition between the Suppliers

There is competition between the various plant collectors at both the source of plants and at the market. As there is little or no cultivation taking place, plant harvesters compete for available plant resources. This competition is exacerbated due to the most accessible plant resources being located in communal areas where property rights are not well defined. This situation leads to competition both within and between different groups, including resident gatherers, contracted gatherers (associated with outside entrepreneurs), and indigenous healers.

There is particular competition in the harvesting of high value species, such as those that are the focus of this survey. As these species are in greatest demand and fetch the highest prices, they are the most sought after trade items. Furthermore, the increasing shortage of high value species results in gatherers, healers and entrepreneurs travelling to more distant locations in order to obtain trade goods.

For example, rural women in northern KwaZulu-Natal now travel into Mozambique to buy Warburgia salutaris bark as local stocks are depleted, creating competition between the Mozambican gatherers, who may be selling to South African or Mozambican buyers.

Apart from competing for plant resources to trade, there is also competition in the sale of plant material to buyers. This competition is associated with trading sites and with customer allegiance. Competition takes place within the street or open markets in Durban and rural markets where products are sold. The gatherers who sell on the streets are generally more mobile and therefore tend to trade more on the periphery of the market, while the more permanent traders have established and maintained their rights to a particular stall site. In order to compete with the more permanent traders, the gatherers may form a group which rotate their visits to the city thereby ensuring that one of the group is always at their market site, maintaining their preferred market position.

There is also competition between street traders and shop traders. Past legislation in South Africa severely limited informal street trading, resulting in the shop traders having a retail monopoly in the medicinal plant industry within urban areas. In the 1980s the shop traders were the main suppliers [Cunningham 1988]. However, this has now changed with the street traders becoming the dominant urban suppliers. The democratization of South Africa and the relaxation of laws limiting informal street trade has resulted in the shop traders losing an estimated 50% to 60% of the medicinal plant market to the street traders. In order to avoid competition on the streets, some gatherers sell plants directly to shop traders and healers developing consumer allegiance for their products. For example, the Durban healers indicated that apart from buying on the street markets, they also had on average five gatherers collecting plants for them.

The Demand for Indigenous Medicines

The demand for indigenous medicines and services is considerable, relative to the demand for western health care services. The black population in Durban indicated that they relied on both health care systems, with 60% of the health care services demanded coming from western health care systems and 40% of the services demanded coming from indigenous medicine. As indigenous medicine is based almost entirely on the use of indigenous plants, a massive demand is generated in terms of both number and mass of plants used.

The value of raw products consumed is considerable. In KwaZulu-Natal, the value of the trade in raw products are worth US$ 13 million (R 60 million) a year, around one-third of the value of the annual maize harvest in the province (one of the largest crops in the province). Households were estimated to be spending between 4% to 8% of their annual incomes on indigenous medicine services.

The demand for medicinal plants is likely to remain buoyant in the future. Consumers indicated that indigenous medicine was not an inferior good and demand is unlikely to decline should income levels and welfare increase in the future. On the contrary, urban consumers indicated that indigenous medicine was more expensive than the subsidized western health services provided by the government, yet they reported that they would be likely to either maintain or increase the frequency of use in the future.

Consumers also indicated that western medicine was not an alternative to indigenous medicine and that irrespective of price, they would have to continue to use indigenous medicine. There are a wide range of ailments and needs which cannot be adequately addressed by western medicine. This implies that indigenous medicine is a basic consumer good, essential for the welfare of black households.

The AIDS pandemic in the region, and the growing international demand for South African medicinal products, is likely to increase the demand for indigenous medicine products in the future.

This market study has been pioneering in terms of developing a broad understanding of consumer demand, showing that there has been considerable ignorance regarding the demand for indigenous medicine and the associated plants in

South Africa. This indicates that South African society has failed to openly discuss and develop a thorough understanding of the demand for indigenous medicine. Consequently, there has been little investment at a formal level in society to address any issues associated with consumer demand.

The Supply of Indigenous Medicines

The indigenous medicine market is based on indigenous plants which are generally harvested from wild plant stocks throughout the province and within the broader region, including neighbouring provinces and other countries. The plant stocks and the harvesting of these stocks are not managed and little cultivation takes place. The combination of high demand and the lack of any significant resource management or production, has resulted in a decline in the available plant stocks.

A wide range of plant species is showing indications of unsustainable use, with the size of the products decreasing, distances to stocks increasing, supply becoming increasingly irregular, and/or some plants becoming unavailable in certain markets. Some popular plants have become extinct outside of protected areas in the province. The supply of indigenous medicinal plants is clearly not sustainable with the current harvesting strategies.

The scarcity of popular plants has led to their under-supply in the market, with considerable increases in product prices, imports into the province, and the use of substitute plants. In addition, there has been an increase in the application of destructive harvesting techniques, which aim at maximizing the harvest from the declining plant stocks in order to maintain income levels in the short term. The supply of popular plant products to the market is declining.

There are however options for sustaining the supply of plants to markets. There are extensive areas of grasslands, woodlands and thickets on private property that have not been intensively harvested in the past. With effective management, these areas could supply a range of products to the markets in the long term. However, the volumes of plant resources available and the harvesting strategies which may be applied need to be investigated. In terms of forest species, there are limited forest areas available and consequently management of existing stocks is unlikely to supply the quantities demanded by the market. In addition, the most popular plants, irrespective of their habitat, exist in such small quantities that management of existing stocks is unlikely to meet market demand.

The cultivation, management and enrichment planting of high value plants is therefore an important strategy to meet consumer demand and to reduce the impacts of the market on biodiversity. The success of cultivation trials undertaken to date have shown good potential for this strategy. Fast-growing species could be supplied in sufficient quantities within a few years. However, the slow-growing popular trees are unlikely to supply the bark quantities demanded in the short term, and alternative products from these plants need to be investigated.

The Marketing of Indigenous Medicinal Plant Products

Over 400 species of plants are marketed in large quantities within KwaZulu-Natal. While the mixing and prescription of plant products is sophisticated, the processing and development of products is extremely limited. There is little processing and value-added to products, with most products sold in the raw form. The most sophisticated product form is a mixture of ground plants. There is little differentiation in product quality and packaging. The entire industry is dominated by simple technology, and by making use of available resources. Most of the value is added when medicines are prescribed by an indigenous healer.

The simple plant products are marketed to consumers, either as self-medication or through healers' prescriptions. The products are marketed within the residential areas dominated by black consumers or in transport nodes throughout urban and rural areas. The conditions in the markets are generally poor, with almost all the consumers indicating that they would prefer more modernized and hygienic conditions. The lack of storage facilities and trading infrastructure frequently results in the spoiling of raw material resulting in wastage and/or a decrease in product quality. Both the healers and consumers have indicated that they are concerned about the quality of the products purchased in these markets.

There is currently no certification of indigenous medicines traded, however, there is a legislation in place which requires the registration of products traded as medicines. The legislation is not currently applied to the indigenous medicine industry due to the informal nature of the trade. This legislation may limit investment in the formal cultivation of plants for the indigenous medicine industry. Unless the current legislation is changed, the production of plants for local markets may have to be limited.

The supply of quality plant products is not only critical for the welfare of millions of consumers, but it is also critical for the welfare of all the people employed in the industry. In KwaZulu-Natal there are between 20 000 and 30 000 people who derive an income trading indigenous plants in some form. Importantly, most of the people involved are black rural women, who are the most marginalized group in South African society. The medicinal plant industry therefore plays a critical role in empowering a large number of rural women.

Overall, the marketing of medicinal plants is poorly developed. Consumers and traders in plant products could benefit considerably through the development of both the products and markets.

Institutional Support for the Marketing of Indigenous Medicinal Plants

In terms of policy support, very little policy has been developed to support the marketing of indigenous plants. Most of the policy has been developed to limit the marketing of plants. There are several regulatory mechanisms (associated with first world standards for medicines and biodiversity priorities) in place but are not being implemented at present. These regulatory mechanisms could however threaten any development emerging from within the industry that may occur with limited resources and which may not meet the required standards of existing legislation. On the other hand, wealthy corporations are unlikely to be as negatively impacted by the existing regulations due to their ability to comply with the high standards stipulated by authorities.

As a result of a largely negative policy environment, there has been insignificant education, training and extension regarding medicinal plant markets. Some efforts have been directed at training market players in the cultivation of medicinal plants but it is insignificant relative to the market size.

Furthermore, most research and development support from government and business has been directed at bio-prospecting and pharmacological investigations, with product development being pursued by major pharmaceutical companies. There are few efforts directed at developing the current markets, their associated products, infrastructure and market players. There is an imbalance in support for indigenous medicine, with most investment directed at seeking commercially useful chemicals within medicinal plants, while little or no investment is being directed to maintain or increase the benefits which the current market is already delivering to society.

The lack of development within the indigenous medicine market in South Africa has also resulted in little information being developed that is useful to the market players. Market information systems are poorly developed, resulting in considerable inefficiency within the markets. Market resources are wasted through inefficient coordination of trade activities. This is particularly problematic given the already short supply of plants and the inability of the current market players to absorb costs.

There is acute competition within the markets and this limits the sharing of knowledge between market players, especially the healers. The lack of sharing limits the development of the indigenous healing profession, with healers largely relying on their own or their mentors' experiences. There is no literature available at present which healers can use as a reference for administering indigenous medicine. One research group in South Africa is presently developing a pharmacopoeia for indigenous medicine. This will help in the development of products for the market by understanding the quantities required for various treatments. However, with over 400 plant species traded, the completion of this task is unlikely to be achieved in the short to medium term.

At the market level, there has been little development due to competition and the under-developed capacity of most market players. With high levels of illiteracy and few business skills, the industry has been unable to develop. In terms of the healers, there are numerous healers' organizations which serve the healers' interests. However, as they focus largely on healing issues, little investment is made at an industry level.

The combination of a negative policy environment and the limited capacity of market players to cooperate and promote their own development has resulted in an industry which is large but grossly underdeveloped.

Opportunities and Constraints in the Medicinal Plant Markets

There are a number of opportunities and constraints which have been identified in the market study. These are summarized below and form the basis for making recommendations for further action in the markets.

The opportunities associated with consumer demand in the indigenous medicine market include:

- strong probability of a growing demand,
- a culturally entrenched demand,
- indigenous medicine is a basic consumer good,
- demand is relatively unresponsive to price changes,
- willingness to pay high prices for more scarce items,
- there are few accepted alternatives,
- consumers prefer better quality products,
- consumers prefer more modem and hygienic packaging, dispensing locations and retail outlets,
- dynamic nature of indigenous medicine and adaptability,
- widespread demand for indigenous medicinal products in African and northern hemisphere countries, and
- different standards required by different consumer groups.

The opportunities on the supply side of the indigenous medicine market include:

- availability of scarce medicinal plants in remote locations,
- availability of medicinal plants on commercial farmlands,
- availability of bark products from logging operations in other parts of South Africa,
- availability of plant supply from changing land-use,
- availability of medicinal plants on managed communal lands,
- availability of a wide range of cultivation, processing, and marketing expertise in other sectors,
- access to international examples of medicine production for traditional markets,
- a large demand for new agricultural opportunities on commercial farms, subsistence farms, and redistributed farms,
- availability of progressive farmers with access to resources,
- robust nature of indigenous medicinal plants which require few agricultural inputs,
- wide range of sites for product distribution, ranging from the farm gate to urban processing factories,
- ability to supply specific species at times of the year when they are usually not available,
- a large number of plant gatherers with appropriate knowledge that could promote the cultivation of plants for the market,
- an established market system that could provide communication mechanisms for any proposed market developments,
- documentation and establishment of accepted guidelines for use and dosages of medicinal plants, and
- several organizations have experience in indigenous medicine markets and in the cultivation of medicinal plant species in farming and nursery systems.

The constraints facing the indigenous medicinal plant market include:

- a policy environment which is negative towards the industry,
- absence of a coherent strategy for transforming the industry into one which is sustainable,
- no government recognition of the opportunities offered by medicinal plants to promote development,
- government departments who may facilitate market development already face severe budget constraints within existing priorities,
- vested interests within existing government departments to maintain the status quo,
- common property or open access rights regimes in large areas which frequently promote resource degradation,
- bureaucratic controls concerning the formal trade of indigenous medicines, which may limit product development to only highly sophisticated operations with massive financial resources,
- a narrow perspective of indigenous medicine in academia, business and government,
- an industry with aggressive competition within and between market segments, resulting in the industry having limited lobbying ability,
- competition which is likely to increase and reduce returns for the lower end of the market,
- competition within the industry that undermines rather than develops the industry,
- an almost total reliance on wild harvested plants for the trade,
- declining plant populations which results in many high value species becoming increasingly inaccessible,
- diminishing product development opportunities due to limited access to sufficient plant stocks,
- local extinctions are resulting in a decline in the genetic variation within high value species,

- supply of plant products is irregular, in quantity and quality,
- forest resources are extremely limited and will provide few of the scarce species in the future,
- there are few production initiatives in the province,
- many high value species are slow-growing,
- literacy of a large number of market players is poor, creating limitations for developing the industry,
- business skills are poorly developed in a number of the sectors,
- there are few skills in the sustainable use of medicinal plant resources,
- there are inefficient market information sharing systems in the industry,
- there is little knowledge of the financial opportunities in cultivating and managing stocks of medicinal plant species,
- lack of information regarding financial feasibility discourages financing institutions from supplying credit,
- there is little known of the condition of plant stocks on privately owned farms,
- distances between major markets and various plant sources are large, generating large costs in the trade, and
- research funds are directed at bioprospecting, with few resources focused on developing the existing industry.

Potential Future Scenarios for the Medicinal Plant Industry

There are a number of scenarios which could develop in the South African indigenous medicinal plant markets, depending on the relationship between a range of fixed and variable factors in the market. The fixed factors include:

- a large and growing local and international demand for medicinal plants,
- a declining supply of forest species in the short term,
- a fluctuating supply of grassland and savannah species in the short term,

- an increase in the price of scarce plants,
- diverse cultivation potential of indigenous medicinal plants,
- an increase in the number and diversity of market players,
- a negative policy environment in the short term, and
- majority of the current market players having limited business skills in the short term.

In contrast to the fixed factors, there are variable factors which will, to a large extent, determine how the market will change in the future. The key variable factors are driven by the actions of the different market players and the associated authorities. The variable actions of these key players include:

- degree to which the current market players cooperate to develop a common vision and to lobby for government support,
- responses of government departments (Health, Agriculture, Trade and Industry, and Environment and Tourism) to the indigenous medicine industry,
- responses of national, provincial, and local political leaders to the indigenous medicine industry,
- response of formal business to the opportunities in the industry, and
- quantities demanded for different levels of processing, certification, standards, and packaging.

The study identified three potential scenarios which could develop depending on the actions of key role players in the markets. The possible scenarios are as follows.

Scenario 1—No intervention the continuation of the status quo - where there is limited investment in promoting the supply of popular plants to the current market players. Consequently, large commercial interests are likely to cultivate high value plants and trade processed products, while most of the current market players continue to compete for a decreasing share to a declining stock of popular plants. A narrow range of species would be cultivated, processed, and distributed for the upper end of the market with a small number of large business interests benefiting. Biodiversity and health care would be negatively impacted.

Scenario 2—Industry driven intervention - collaboration between progressive current market players and skilled business interests is likely to offer large benefits to large and intermediate companies and to a limited number of current market players. Cultivation, processing, and distribution would occur for the middle and upper end of the market. Small-scale traders and gatherers are likely to continue to trade in wild plants, but supply is likely to decline as the consumption of cheap products continues at the lower end of the market. Biodiversity and health care would be negatively impacted.

Scenario 3—Collaborative intervention - collaboration between current market players, government and business interests-this could see the development of a wide range of processed products from simple rural products to sophisticated industrial products. Numerous market players could develop a range of different quality products for a wide range of consumers, with different prices suited the consumers' budgets. Such a scenario, is likely to promote the growth of the industry, and promote development at a broad scale. Investment in resource management is also more likely in this scenario. Health care would also benefit.

The most likely scenario to develop without market interventions is number 2, where big business enters the market and leads market development to suit its own objectives. Current investments by both government and big business are supporting the development of this scenario. Furthermore, current legislation supports the development of the corporate sector by excluding the less developed market players from producing more commercialized indigenous plant products. The costs of this scenario will be borne largely by the current consumers who will lose access to basic consumer goods through price increases and scarcity, and market players will lose access to trade products.

As the current consumers and current market players are largely from the least developed sector of South African society, it is essential to initiate market interventions which promote the welfare of the current consumers and market players, especially at the lower end of the market. At the same time, the opportunities for large-scale corporate involvement at the upper end of the market and in international markets, should be developed. To maximize the benefits to the greatest number of beneficiaries, South Africa needs to focus on achieving the development of both the existing market players and corporate entrants.

The development of the indigenous medicine market in South Africa will promote economic growth, people's development, consumer welfare, and biodiversity conservation. However, this will only be achieved if development takes place across the whole spectrum of the market, from rural resource management and production through to corporate bioprospecting and marketing.

The challenge facing the South African community is to capitalize on the market opportunities and to overcome the market constraints in the medicinal plant industry through achieving a greater balance in the distribution of development resources in public and private sector.

International Trade in Medicinal Plants

There is large-scale international trade in medicinal plants, used both for herbal medicine and for the manufacture of pharmaceutical drugs. There is also growing interest in obtaining samples of plant material, or traditional knowledge about plant uses, to explore for new commercial medical products. The scale of international trade in medicinal plants is difficult to assess, because of a paucity of reliable statistics and trade secrecy, but it is growing rapidly.

Conservation issues in international trade in medicinal plants for existing products mainly concern those plants which are harvested from the 'wild', which is the case for the great majority of species. Conservation issues arise if the trade threatens conservation of biodiversity or is not sustainable. Biodiversity may be threatened if the trade endangers survival of the species, erodes its genetic diversity or causes loss or degradation of important natural or semi-natural ecosystems.

The international movement of plant samples (or traditional knowledge about the uses of plants) for analysis to discover possible new commercial products raises the issue of equitable distribution of rewards in the event of successful commercialisation. Following the Biodiversity Treaty, there is an urgent need for equitable partnerships to be developed between those involved in developing new commercial products from plants and those responsible for conservation of biodiversity (often in the South).

Botanic gardens have long been involved with both medicinal plants and plant movements, but not with conservation. Notable features of botanic gardens relevant to conservation include the fact that they are often major centres of expertise about plants, that they have collections of living plants and that sometimes they have been assigned legal roles concerning the movements of plants between countries (*e.g.* as scientific authorities for CITES). There is also the possibility of botanical gardens being involved in ex situ conservation of plants, as part of integrated conservation strategies aimed at particular plant species. Thus, botanical gardens have special opportunities and responsibilities in respect of conservation issues raised by the international trade in medicinal plants.

If existing trade in medicinal plants results in conservation problems, for example if plants are being over-harvested from wild populations, then potential solutions include the design and implementation of new methods of managing wild populations, or transferring the business to reliance on cultivated plants. Many botanic gardens, having skills in plant propagation and horticulture, are in a special position to assist with the process of introducing plants into cultivation, but they will generally need to work closely with other agencies better equipped to deal with other necessary aspects, including social and economic ones. Success in making harvesting of species sustainable must involve the social dimension.

Botanic gardens are being approached by commercial interests that are interested in developing new medical products, in order to supply plant material, or knowledge about the uses of plants, for testing the development of new products. Botanic gardens are attractive agencies for commercial firms to approach, because of their concentration of botanical expertise. Botanists, for example, may be contracted to collect plant material from the 'wild'. The living collections of botanic gardens may be sampled without the bother of mounting expeditions to, perhaps distant, climes. Botanic gardens, therefore, have a special responsibility to ensure that they only supply samples to commercial interests for evaluation of possible new products under agreements which are ethically just.

International Trade in Medicinal Plants

It has been said that as many as 35 000-70 000 species of plants have been used at one time or another for medicinal purposes (Farnsworth & Soejarto 1991). By far the greater number of species is employed in herbal medicine and is used in unrefined or semi-processed form, often in mixtures which sometimes also contain non-botanical ingredients. A few species are the sources of defined compounds used in the pharmaceutical industry. The overall quantities of plants used medically, in one way or another, are large. Farnsworth and Soejarto (1991), quoting other papers by Farnsworth, state that approximately one-quarter of all prescriptions dispensed from community pharmacies in the USA contain one or more ingredients derived from higher plants.

In many tropical and sub-tropical countries, as in Africa and South and East Asia, the majority of people resort to herbal medicine for the majority of their primary healthcare needs. There are also strong traditions of herbal medicine in parts of Europe, such as Germany, France and eastern Europe generally. The herbal sector is growing fast, increasing by 12-15% by value per year in the UK, USA and Italy (Abrahams 1992). According to a review of a recent consultancy report by McAlpine Thorpe and Warrier (1992), there are more than 2000 herbal medical companies in Europe and more than 220 in the USA; this review states that Germany is the largest market in the world for herbal medicines, with annual sales of $1.2 billion representing nearly 25% of the national pharmaceutical market. The USA is the next largest market with sales of $480 million.

It is difficult to obtain precise information about the structure and scale of the international trade in medicinal plants. Anna Lewington, who recently carried out a short-term study on behalf of WWF of the importation of medicinal plants into Europe and attendant conservation problems, found trade statistics and customs records to be very inadequate, and the industry as a whole not particularly forthcoming about its activities (Lewington 1992a). A complication in some cases is that there can be no clear distinction between medicinal, food, spice and aromatic plants.

The most recent report available to the general public dealing with European imports appears to be by the International Trade Centre, Geneva, in 1982. This report states that 8 countries then belonging to the EEC imported 80 738 tons of 'vegetation plant materials used in pharmacy' in 1980, the biggest importer being Germany with 31 452 tons, followed by France. Quantities will certainly be larger now, as it is widely acknowledged that the trade has grown. Lewington (1992a) estimates that 500, and possibly as many as 600, species of medicinal plants are traded through Hamburg, Germany, which lies at the heart of the import business in Europe. In 1980 India was the biggest exporter of medicinal plants to Europe (10 055 tons out of the 80 738 imported). Eastern Europe is another important source of supply.

Major international trade in medicinal plants is not only from developing to urban-industrial countries. For instance, there is major trade from the Himalayas, including Nepal, to India and beyond, mostly for use in herbal medicine (notably ayurvedic medicine). The volume of this trade is unknown, because it is believed that the greater part of it passes through unofficial channels. Unregulated harvesting of medicinal plants in the Himalayas is a cause for conservation concern.

The majority of conservation problems that result from existing trade in medicinal plants arise if the plants are 'wild' collected, as opposed to being cultivated. Lewington (1992a) reports that it is very difficult to determine the precise origin of medicinal plants currently imported into Europe, a complicating factor being that some species which are cultivated are also collected to some extent from the wild. Judging by Lewington (1992a) and various articles in Akerele et al. (1991), only a few species, required in large quantities, are cultivated to any significant extent. The great majority of species in international trade, certainly most of those which are used in herbal medicine, are harvested in the wild.

Case Study: Prunus Africana

Information has been compiled by WWF on conservation issues associated with international trade in Prunus africana for medicinal products (Lewington 1992b). Prunus africana is a large and widely distributed tree of wet montane forests in Africa. Extracts of the bark, marketed as Tadenon (France) and Pigenil (Italy), are used in several European countries to treat early stages of benign prostatic hypertrophy.

The use of this medicine first came to the attention of European industry from the earlier traditional employment of the bark in warm milk in South Africa to treat "old man's disease". Prunus africana is, in fact, a widely used medicinal plants in many parts of Africa. Today, bark, or extracts from the bark, are exported to Europe in significant quantities from Cameroon, Zaire (Kivu), Kenya and Madagascar. So far as can be determined, all harvesting is from uncultivated 'wild' trees growing in forests. It is difficult to establish the scale of the trade, but our information indicates that the total harvest of wet bark each year might be in the order of 1600-2000 tonnes. We estimate that the total value of the trade at the point of sale in European pharmacies as over $100 million a year, a figure which can be compared with the amount received by all those collectors who gain some income from the harvesting of the bark in Africa, estimated in total at less than $200 000 a year.

The manner of collection of Prunus bark, at least in Cameroon and Zaire, seems to be similar to the way many plants are harvested from the 'wild', all over the world for the international medicinal plant trade. Businessmen or their agents contract local villagers for collection of the plant material which is required; this material is then more or less indiscriminately harvested from surrounding areas. A variant, reported in the case of collection of medicinal plants in the Himalayas, is for merchants to bring in their own labourers to the collecting area from elsewhere. It is difficult for poor people to resist this chance of an income, however small it may be, even if they are aware that the long-term effects may be disadvantageous.

Conservation issues associated with Prunus collection are that the bark is being harvested unsustainably, that it is causing degradation and in some cases loss of an important ecosystem (wet montane forest - vital for catchment protection in Africa) and that it is almost certainly eroding genetic diversity within Prunus africana. There is no threat to survival of the species as such (as seems often to be the case with collection of medicinal plants traded internationally).

The Prunus issue first came to the attention of WWF in Cameroon, where indiscriminate harvesting has destroyed many trees in a small remnant montane forest on West Africa's second highest mountain, Mt Kilum. According to local sources, the harvesting has also been indirectly responsible for triggering total forest loss, associated with the sudden injection of a heavy dose of materialistic values, undermining local traditions which afforded some protection to the forests.

Conservation Issues Relating to Trade in Medicinal Plants for Existing Products

Trade in medicinal plants for established products can be considered to result in conservation issues if the trade:

- Endangers survival of the species;
- Seriously erodes genetic diversity of the species;
- Threatens the survival or functional integrity of important natural or semi-natural ecosystems;
- Is non-sustainable, which in its most basic form, means that the species is extracted from a particular site at a rate greater than that at which it is being replaced.

Conservation Issues and the Development of New Products

There seems to be an increasing interest by natural product chemists and the pharmaceutical industry in exploring the plant world for possible new medical products. Plants have contributed much to modern Western medicine, in a number of different ways (Hollman 1991): (1) purified compounds from plants are used directly as medicines (*e.g.* morphine from the opium poppy Papaver somniferum), (2) compounds are extracted from plants and then used in a modified form (*e.g.* steroid drugs from Dioscorea), (3) an active principle in the plant has provided the stimulus to produce new medicines by total synthesis (*e.g.* the synthetic drug Intal developed from investigations based on Ammi visnaga), and (4) the mode of action of a plant medicine has been copied to provide a better synthetic drug (muscle relaxants from curare). New biotechnologies will open up new ways in which plants can contribute to advances in medicine.

Strategies for choosing which plants to investigate in the search for new medical products include the random selection of plants based on taxonomic affinity, or the pursuit of leads based on ethnobotanical knowledge. The use of plants in folk medicine has led to the discovery of the majority of major drugs used in Western medicine with an origin in plants (Hollman 1991). Traditional knowledge, accumulated through years of experience, can be regarded as the product of a natural screening process.

The search for new medical products based on plants often involves the movement of plant samples or information about plants between countries, and thus is a type of plant trade (see Fig 2). Differences with trade for products which already exist are: (1) the amount of material involved is generally very much smaller; (2) the transfer of material or information may only occur once or, perhaps only a few times (an initial sample for screening; larger quantities for product development); (3) there is a high chance that no commercial products will result and (4), if commercial success does eventually result, then profits may be very large (due to a monopoly position protected by patenting during early years of marketing of a new pharmaceutical drug).

The sizes of samples required for initial screening are generally small, but sometimes larger quantities are needed for follow-up testing; this can result in serious depletion of plant populations. An example is the collection of Dioscorea deltoides, allegedly for German pharmaceutical firms, in the Khasi and nearby hills in India in the 1980s, allegedly resulting in local near-extinction. This plant is traditionally used in the area as a female contraceptive, so that, ironically, it is possible that advances in the development of contraceptive drugs in Europe have been instrumental in removing the availability of a traditionally used means of contraception from another part of the world.

The most pressing conservation issue in the discovery and commercialisation of new plant-derived or plant-inspired products (including medicines) is the question of how to create equitable partnerships, in order to return a proportion of profits deriving from commercialisation back to the country of origin of the species, plant material or knowledge about the species.

Medicinal Plants: the Historical Role of Botanic Gardens

A botanic garden has been defined as 'a garden containing scientifically ordered and maintained collections of plants, usually documented and labelled, and open to the public for the purposes of recreation, education and research' (Botanic Gardens Conservation Secretariat (BGCI) 1989). Botanic gardens have a long history of involvement with medicinal plants and with movements of plants around the globe, but not with conservation. According to Heywood (1991), the first botanic gardens in the western tradition, at Pisa, Padua and Florence in Italy, were medicinal plant gardens attached to medical faculties or schools. There is also a long link between medicine and the garden in Asia. At the famous cultural site of Sigiriya in Sri Lanka, dating from the fifth century AD, excavation has revealed the well preserved remains of very extensive, formally laid out, pleasure gardens, and historic records indicate that there was once also a garden for medicinal plants.

The expansion of European power around the world from the fifteenth century onwards was followed by a wave of creation of botanic gardens and arboreta in the tropics and subtropics. These gardens were established principally for economic evaluation of plants for the benefit of the colonial powers.

Heywood (1991) states that medicinal plants were given little emphasis by these gardens and arboreta, but nevertheless they did play important roles in introducing tea, coffee and Cola to new areas (all these species can be considered medicinal plants) and also introductions of quinine.

The first potential crop tried out at Hakgala Botanic Garden in Sri Lanka was quinine (in 1861), soon followed by tea (in 1865). The latter was successful, and was followed by development of a major industry.

Many plants, both those which had been previously domesticated and those which had not, were transported around the globe and tried out in botanic gardens or arboreta in the colonies. For example, the Germans established a botanic garden at Amani in the East Usambara (Tanzania) in 1902, planting about 900 species, nearly all exotics and nearly all woody. The Royal Botanic Gardens Kew at one time had a policy of facilitating the movement of plants around the British Empire.

From a modern conservation perspective, the historical role of botanic gardens in facilitating plant movements can be seen to have had some unfortunate consequences, both as regards natural ecosystems and mental attitudes:

- Some species introduced by botanic gardens have proved invasive and a serious threat to natural ecosystems. Many serious problems of plant invasion on oceanic islands originated from introductions made by botanic gardens. A gardener from Kew, for example, was dispatched to St Helena to introduce quinine Cinchona officinalis, intended as a cash crop: "The cultivation of this valuable plant... has been undertaken on the south side of the high central ridge of the Island. The undertaking was commenced five years ago under such favourable auspices, and promised such success, that it is much to be regretted that the experiment was not continued. In the year 1871 there were three hundred plants of this species growing amongst the native vegetation. The first Cinchona plant ever raised in the island was from seed sent from the Royal Gardens at Kew in 1866-7" (Melliss 1875). The Cinchona industry never became established on St Helena, but Cinchona is still quite abundant as an invasive exotic element in the native vegetation.

An example of a serious plant invasion from a continental botanical garden is the invasion of endemic-rich tropical forest on the East Usambara by Maesopsis eminii, originally introduced in the Amani Botanic Garden. Maesopsis is a serious threat to the maintenance of biological diversity and good catchment properties (Hamilton & Bensted Smith 1989). Maesopsis is not alone: there are several other exotic species invading the Usambara forests, many originating from plantings in the botanic garden.

- The emphasis on moving plants around the world in a free and easy manner seems to have often helped to foster an unstated attitude that exotic plants are somehow superior to local plants, not only for planting for forestry products, but also as crops. Of course, there are some species and cultivars with outstanding properties which may merit growing on very extensive scales, but promotion of a few favoured genera or species, such as Eucalyptus in forestry and 'modern' varieties of crops has been a factor in reducing biodiversity in ecosystems worldwide. Many local landraces of crops have been lost through the introduction of modern cultivars, resulting in serious loss of valuable germplasm. Modern varieties may have their advantages, but they also have disadvantages, involving susceptibility to diseases and/or pests and creation of a dependency on high inputs of fertilisers and pesticides, which in many situations, cannot be economically maintained and which can increase economic inequality.
- The cavalier manner in which plants have been moved around the world during the last five hundred years has tended to result in a mental attitude which sees all 'wild' plants and 'traditional' varieties of crops, as well as local knowledge about the uses of plants as medicines and for other purposes, as common global property. This contrasts with the promotion of plant breeder rights in respect of

the values of new crop varieties, which give a form of patent protection to plant breeders. Biodiversity and traditional knowledge about plants have become undervalued.

Recent years have seen the rise of many large industries operating internationally: some of these are involved in exploring plants for new medicinal products. These industries are strongly motivated by profit and are based overwhelmingly in Western countries. Many of these industries have research capabilities far beyond those of most governments in developing countries, and their activities will undoubtedly dominate the search for new medicines from plants in the future. These industries are likely to regard botanic gardens as resources which, in certain situations, are worthy of exploitation. Botanic gardens have several commodities which these companies need: expertise in identifying plants, expertise in collecting plant material of required types from the 'wild' and easy sources of supply of plant material from living collections or dried specimens. Their use avoids all the costs and difficulties of mounting expeditions to, perhaps, distant countries.

How can Botanic Gardens Contribute to Conservation of Medicinal Plants in International Trade?

Some desirable conservation activities to combat conservation problems arising from the international trade in medicinal plants. Some of these activities are suitable for botanic gardens which have a number of special features which give them certain advantages and also convey on them certain responsibilities in this area. The ability of botanic gardens to become involved in conservation of medicinal plants depends partly on their available resources, which vary greatly from garden to garden.

If medicinal plants are being over-harvested from the 'wild', then it is possible that collection is not only not sustainable, but also that the genetic diversity of the species is being eroded and that natural ecosystems are being degraded. Except where there is a strong sense of community solidarity, it is likely to be often difficult to develop sustainable harvesting based on community control alone, given that collection of 'wild' medicinal plants for sale is often undertaken essentially competitively. The successful implementation of ways of harvesting 'wild' plants sustainably is generally likely to involve agencies such as forest departments, probably usually working closely with local people.

Encouragement of cultivation is often likely to be useful, in order to take the pressure off wild stocks, thus helping to conserve genetic diversity and perhaps being a more reliable source of income for village people. Clearly botanic gardens, with their expertise in gardening and other botanical disciplines, can often play useful roles in helping to select and develop varieties for cultivation, and in undertaking research on techniques for propagation and cultivation.

Where the aim is to produce sustainability in supply of plant material for the manufacture of medicines (as will often be the case), then assessments of whether sustainability has been achieved through the introduction of cultivation must consider both the social and ecological dimensions. If over-harvesting of plant material from the 'wild' by a poor rural community is replaced by cultivation by rich farmers, then it cannot be said that sustainability has been achieved, in terms of the total socio-ecological system.

Botanic gardens can also have a role to play in the conservation of genetic diversity within species of medicinal plants. In general, genetic diversity should be conserved through conservation of a network of in situ populations which together reasonably cover the total genetic diversity of the species. Usually these populations will be on land owned by other organisations or private individuals, not botanical gardens.

However, botanical gardens may have a role to play in helping to develop back-up facilities for ex situ conservation of threatened medicinal plants. This could be through providing expertise to land-holding agencies or individuals for the development of small nurseries at each in situ site, so as to propagate the species and reintroduce them into nature where populations are low. Possibly, botanic gardens could also assist through the development of germplasm banks such as seed collections, though medicinal plants are not high on the list of ex situ conservation programmes of this type at present. Botanic gardens have a major responsibility for ensuring that arrangements are equitable in cases where they have some involvement in providing plant samples or information about plants to commercial interests for investigation for new products.

Botanic gardens are therefore in the front-line of implementing the principles of the Biodiversity Treaty discussed in Brazil in June 1992. The Biodiversity Treaty will presumably eventually result in new national legislation concerning the exploitation of plant diversity and the requirements for rewards from commercialisation. Botanists and ethnobotanists, including those associated with botanic gardens, will have to observe this legislation, but they have the additional responsibility, in any case, to ensure that their behaviour is ethical. Unfortunately there is little experience of suitable agreements between suppliers of plant material or information about plants and commercial interests.

As far as I know, there are no cases in which such agreements have been followed by the successful commercialisation of new products, and then by the actual return of just rewards to sources. It is doubtful whether any very strict conservation guidelines can be written at the present time, given the lack of practical experience, but WWF, through Dr. Anthony Cunningham, is in the process of preparing general guidelines for botanists and ethnobotanists to indicate the parameters of the issue and to assist them in arriving at fair arrangements. We hope to have these guidelines ready by the end of December 1992.

7

Sustainable Use of Medicinal Plants

Wild plants have been an important component of healthcare throughout human history. Medicinal plants continue to make important contributions to healthcare and livelihoods, and were recently identified by FAO as being among the most valuable non-wood forest products (FAO, 1999). Unfortunately, harvests to meet the demand for a growing number of medicinal species are in many cases exceeding sustainable levels. Wild medicinal plant populations and the benefits derived therefrom are coming under threat as a result.

More effective co-operation among the variety of institutions concerned with the use and trade of medicinal plants, including those from the healthcare, conservation, development and commercial sectors, is required to ensure the conservation of biodiversity and continued availability of medicinal resources.

Medicinal Plants and Health

Medicinal plants underpin healthcare practices across the globe. Much of the world's population depends on traditional medicine to meet daily health requirements, especially within developing countries. Traditional medicine in turn relies heavily on medicinal plants. Reliance on natural medicinal resources can be attributed to cultural preferences as well as to the high cost and inaccessibility of western medicine.

Use of plant-based remedies is also widespread in many industrialised countries. Herbal remedies are made directly from plant materials, and numerous pharmaceutical products are based on or derived from plant compounds. Similarly, cosmetics and other household products may contain plants of medicinal or therapeutic value. The use of medicinal plants for healthcare is believed to be increasing throughout much of the world, *e.g.* in Africa (Cunningham, 1993; Marshall, 1998), China (He and Sheng, 1997), Europe (Lange, 1998) and North America (Brevoort, 1998).

Commercial Trade in Medicinal Plants

The large and growing demand for plant-based medicines and changing population patterns have prompted a growing domestic and international trade in medicinal plants. The following information from Lange (1997, 1998) gives an indication of the scale of the trade.

According to Customs data, approximately 440 000 t of medicinal and aromatic plants were traded internationally in 1996, with a reported value of USD1.3 billion. Hong Kong, Japan and Germany were the largest importers during 1994 and 1995, the United States being the third largest importer overall during the period 1992 to 1996. Approximately 60% of imports into Germany in 1996 originated from non-European countries, with exports from Asia dominating the trade, followed by exports from Africa. China was also by far the largest exporter of medicinal and aromatic plants to world markets during the mid-1990s, with average exports topping 140 000 t from 1992 to 1996. The second largest exporter was India, with export volumes averaging approximately 36 000 t during this period.

A wide diversity of medicinal plant species are used and traded for medicinal purposes. A recent TRAFFIC 1 study of the European medicinal plant trade (Lange, 1998) estimates that over 2000 medicinal and aromatic plant species are used commercially in Europe, of which 1200 to 1300 are native. Approximately 90% of the European species are collected from the wild, with eastern Europe and the Mediterranean regions being the main suppliers (Lange, 1998). In India it has been estimated that approximately 7500 species are used for medicinal and veterinary purposes (Uniyal et al., 2000). Over 10,000 species are used medicinally in China (He and Cheng,

1991), with 1,000 species commonly used in medicinal preparations, of which 80% are wild-collected (He and Sheng, 1997).

Harvest of medicinal plants to supply domestic and foreign markets provides an important source of cash income in many countries. In Nepal, for example, Olsen (1998, cited in Olsen, 1999) has estimated that 470 000 households are engaged in commercial collection of medicinal plants. Several publications in the FAO Non-Wood Forest Product Series have drawn attention to the current and potential role of medicinal plants in economic development.

Declines in Medicinal Plant Populations

There is growing evidence that the populations of many medicinal plant species are declining in the wild. These declines are the result of several factors, key among them being habitat degradation and expanding harvests. TRAFFIC's study of the European medicinal plant trade identified approximately 150 European species reported to be threatened in at least one European country (Lange, 1998); a TRAFFIC study in East/ Southern Africa identified approximately 100 species of conservation concern in one or more countries (Marshall, 1998). Reviews of the status of medicinal plant species according to the 'Red List' (threat) criteria of IUCN-The World Conservation Union in three regions of India identified approximately 70 species considered at risk (Anon., 1998).

Fourteen species have been included in the Appendices of the Convention on International Trade in Endangered Species of Wild Fauna and Flora (CITES) owing to concern that they might be threatened unless international trade is subject to specific controls.

A Multi-sectoral Challenge

A variety of individuals and institutions have an interest in securing the future of medicinal plant species both because of the direct benefits they provide and in the wider context of biodiversity conservation. These range from local collectors, healers and communities to national governments, multinational corporations, non-governmental organisations and international treaty bodies. Areas of concern include the role of medicinal plants in healthcare (both local and national) and development, biodiversity conservation, the use of traditional knowledge, intellectual property rights and benefit sharing, marketing and trade.

Individuals acting within different sectors are frequently unaware of the shared and/or conflicting interests and motivations of other sectors. In some cases, this can lead to different sectors unnecessarily working at cross-purposes. For example, government agencies charged with species conservation may be unaware of the importance accorded medicinal plants by health agencies. Similarly, health agencies may be unaware of the status of certain species in the wild. The former may seek to restrict use and trade of specific species, while the latter seeks to expand it.

In many cases, the long-term interests sought by different sectors might be better served through increased information sharing, dialogue and cooperation. For example, efforts to promote commercial trade of medicinal plants as a basis for economic development would benefit from greater knowledge of species biology and market dynamics. Efforts to ensure the conservation of medicinal plant species and their availability for healthcare would similarly benefit from such knowledge. Policies intended to support these and/or other objectives similarly seem more likely to succeed if the full range of stakeholder perspectives and interests are understood and taken into account.

The need for more effective cross-sector collaboration to address medicinal plant conservation issues was first brought to world attention by the International Consultation on the Conservation of Medicinal Plants, convened by the World Wide Fund for Nature (WWF), IUCN and the World Health Organisation in Chiang Mai, Thailand, in 1988. This message was reiterated a decade later during the international conference Medicinal Plants for Survival, hosted by the Foundation for Revitalization of Local Health Traditions in Bangalore, India in 1998. More recently, 20 participants at the symposium

Medicinal Utilisation of Wild Species signed a 'Joint Declaration for the Health of People and Nature', which emphasises the need to address conservation concerns in a multi-disciplinary and collaborative manner. Signatories include representatives of the phytopharmaceutical industry, practitioners' associations and conservation organisations.

The depository for the Joint Declaration is WWF Germany, who organised the symposium with TRAFFIC Europe—Germany, and, who, with TRAFFIC, is working to encourage and monitor the Declaration's transformation from words into actions.

These and other initiatives indicate the potential for more and more effective cooperation among individuals and institutions concerned with the use, trade and conservation of medicinal plants. Additional effort needs to be invested in putting these good intentions into practice in order to secure the future of medicinal plant populations and the benefits they provide.

Developing the Medicinal Plants

The medicinal properties of plant species have made an outstanding contribution in the origin and evolution of many traditional herbal therapies. These traditional knowledge systems have started to disappear with the passage of time due to scarcity of written documents and relatively low income in these traditions.

Over the past few years, however, the medicinal plants have regained a wide recognition due to an escalating faith in herbal medicine in view of its lesser side effects compared to allopathic medicine in addition the necessity of meeting the requirements of medicine for an increasing human population. Through the realization of the continuous erosion of traditional knowledge of plants used for medicine in the past and the renewed interest at the present time, a need existed to review this valuable knowledge of medicinal plants with the purpose of developing medicinal plants sectors across the different states in India. Our major objectives therefore were to explore the potential in medicinal plants resources, to understand the challenges and opportunities with the medicinal plants sector, and also to suggest recommendations based upon the present state of knowledge for the establishment and smooth functioning of the medicinal plants sector along with improving the living standards of the underprivileged communities.

The review reveals that northern India harbours a rich diversity of valuable medicinal plants, and attempts are being made at different levels for sustainable utilization of this resource in order to develop the medicinal plants sector.

Background

Forests have played key roles in the lives of people living in both mountains and lowland areas by supplying fresh water and oxygen as well as providing a diversity of valuable forest products for food and medicine. The age-old traditional values attached with the various forest types and the varieties of forest products (*i.e.*, medicinal plants) have gained tremendous importance in the present century.

Furthermore, the cosmetic industries are increasingly using natural ingredients in their products, and these natural ingredients include extracts of several medicinal plants. India and China are two of the largest countries in Asia, which have the richest arrays of registered and relatively well-known medicinal plants. Since the Indian subcontinent is well known for its diversity of forest products and the age-old healthcare traditions, there is an urgent need to establish these traditional values in both the national and international perspectives realizing the ongoing developmental trends in traditional knowledge.

Apart from health care, medicinal plants are mainly the alternate income-generating source of underprivileged communities; therefore, strengthening this sector may benefit and improve the living standard of poor people. A great deal of traditional knowledge of the use of various plant species is still intact with the indigenous people, and this fact is especially relevant with the mountainous areas such as the Himalaya due to less accessibility of terrain and comparatively slow rate of development.

The ongoing growing recognition of medicinal plants is due to several reasons, including escalating faith in herbal medicine. Allopathic medicine may cure a wide range of diseases; however, its high prices and side-effects are causing many people to return to herbal medicines which have fewer side effects.

The instant rising demand of plant-based drugs is unfortunately creating heavy pressure on some selected high-value medicinal plant populations in the wild due to over-harvesting. Several of these medicinal plant species have slow growth rates, low population densities, and narrow geographic ranges; therefore they are more prone to extinction. Conversely, because information on the use of plant species for therapeutic purpose has been passed from one generation to the next through oral tradition, this knowledge of therapeutic plants has started to decline and become obsolete through the lack of recognition by younger generations as a result of a shift in attitude and ongoing socio-economic changes.

Furthermore, the indigenous knowledge on the use of lesser-known medicinal plants is also rapidly declining. Through the realization of the continuous erosion in the traditional knowledge of many valuable plants for medicine in the past and the renewal interest currently, the need existed to review the valuable knowledge with the expectation of developing the medicinal plants sector.

The present paper is therefore concerned with the following major objectives: (1) discovering the role, value, diversity and potential in medicinal plants resources, (2) assessing various aspects of medicinal plant sector, which includes challenges and opportunities, and (3) suggesting recommendations based on existing information for the benefit and development of medicinal plants sector in northern India.

Use and Diversity in Medicinal Plants

In India, of the 17,000 species of higher plants, 7500 are known for medicinal uses. This proportion of medicinal plants is the highest proportion of plants known for their medical purposes in any country of the world for the existing flora of that respective country. Ayurveda, the oldest medical system in Indian sub-continent, has alone reported approximately 2000 medicinal plant species, followed by Siddha and Unani. The Charak Samhita, an age-old written document on herbal therapy, reports on the production of 340 herbal drugs and their indigenous uses. Currently, approximately 25% of drugs are derived from plants, and many others are synthetic analogues built on prototype compounds isolated from plant species in modern pharmacopoeia.

The northern part of India harbours a great diversity of medicinal plants because of the majestic Himalayan range. So far about 8000 species of angiosperms, 44 species of gymnosperms and 600 species of pteridophytes have been reported in the Indian Himalaya, of these 1748 species are known as medicinal plants. The maximum medicinal plants (1717 species) have been reported around the 1800 m elevation range. On the regional scale, the maximum species of medicinal plants have been reported from Uttaranchal, followed by Sikkim and North Bengal. The trans-Himalaya sustains about 337 species of medicinal plants, which is low compared to other areas of the Himalaya due to the distinct geography and ecological marginal conditions .

Several plant species are endemic to the Himalayan region. Out of total known number of higher plants from India, approximately 46% are endemic to the Himalaya. Of the total medicinal plant species, sixty-two species of medicinal plants are endemic to the Himalaya and 208 extend their distribution to the adjacent areas, and are therefore classified as near endemic. Over 200 species of Himalayan medicinal plants are consumed raw, roasted, boiled, fried, cooked, or they are used in the form of oil, spices, jams or pickles.

The indigenous communities use some medicinal plant species as a source of food, fodder, timber as well as various other ethnobotanical purposes. For example, apart from the use of Myrica esculenta and Terminalia bellirica as medicines, the fruits of these species are edible, the leaves are used for fodder and the wood is used for fuel. Approximately 81 species of Himalayan medicinal plants are known to be used for the extraction of oil. Of the total 675 species of Himalayan wild edibles, 171 are used for the treatment of diseases. The crop plants diversity is also a source of traditional medicine .

Apart from the human use, animal husbandry uses many plant species as its primary source of healthcare in northern India. The reliance on medicinal plants is also due to cultural preferences. Medicinal plants have strong acceptance in religious activities of north Indian native communities, who worship the plants in the form of various gods, goddesses and minor deities. Origanum vulgare, Saussurea obvallata, Ocimum sanctum, Cedrus deodara, Cynodon dactylon, Aegle marmelos, Juniperus communis, Musa paradissica, Nardostachys grandiflora, Zanthoxylum armatum, Ficus benghalensis, and Ficus religiosa are examples of the medicinal plants highly used for medicinal as well as a religious purposes by the Hindus in northern India.

The Buddhist community in northern India regards Terminalia chebula as an important medicine as well as sacred fruit. It has been stated long ago that the therapeutic potency of medicinal plants is more effective and better suited to a person of a particular region or culture in which the plant is naturally growing. This idea has given a way to the development of a new drug for heart patients of specific ethnic groups in African countries .

Challenges in Medicinal Plants Sector

The continuous increase in human population is one of the causes for concern in meeting the daily requirements of food and medicine as the economy and livelihoods of human societies living in developing countries primarily depend on forest products. This phenomenon is leading to continuous erosion of forest and the forest products, thus making challenge to meet the requirements as well as to conserve useful bio-resources.

More and more species are being gradually added in the Materia Medica; however, the standards of their purity and correct identification do not keep pace with the process of expansion. The market prices for medicinal plants and derived materials provide only a limited insight into the workings of the market, and not on the precise information of profits, supply and demand. We have identified the following major features and challenges on the basis of examining the existing knowledge on the medicinal plants sector.

Rising Demand

The World Health Organization (WHO) has estimated the present demand for medicinal plants is approximately US $14 billion per year. The demand for medicinal plant-based raw materials is growing at the rate of 15 to 25% annually, and according to an estimate of WHO, the demand for medicinal plants is likely to increase more than US $5 trillion in 2050. In India, the medicinal plant-related trade is estimated to be approximately US $1 billion per year.

The projected escalating demand of medicinal plants has led to the over-harvesting of many plants from wild, which subsequently results in the loss of their existing populations. For example, the large quantity of Himalayan yew (Taxus baccata) has been gathered from the wild since its extract, taxol, was established as a use in the treatment of ovarian cancer. Aconitum heterophyllum, Nardostachys grandiflora, Dactylorhiza hatagirea, Polygonatum verticillatum, Gloriosa superba, Arnebia benthamii and Megacarpoea polyandra are other examples of north Indian medicinal plant species which have been overexploited for therapeutic uses and have subsequently been placed today in rare and endangered categories.

Many medicinal plant species are used in curing more than one disease, and as a result, these species are under pressure due to over collection from wild. For example, Hemidesmus indicus is used to cure 34 types of diseases; Aegle marmelos 31, Phyllanthus emblica 29, and Gloriosa superba 28. Over-exploitation and continuous depletion of medicinal plants have not only affected their supply and loss of genetic diversity, but have seriously affected the livelihoods of indigenous people living in the forest margins .

More than 95% of the 400 plant species used in preparing medicine by various industries are harvested from wild populations in India. Harvesting medicinal plants for commercial use, coupled with the destructive harvest of underground parts of slow reproducing, slow growing and habitat-specific species, are the crucial factors in meeting the goal of sustainability. Harvesting shoots and leaves of medicinal plants may decline their photosynthetic capacity, and as well as the potential for survival and effective propagation. Medicinal plants tolerance to harvest varies with climatic conditions as the temperate herbs become highly vulnerable to harvest of individuals. Furthermore, rising demand with shrinking habitats may lead to the local extinction of many medicinal plant species.

Increasing Rarity

The continuous exploitation of several medicinal plant species from the wild and substantial loss of their habitats during past 15 years have resulted in population decline of many high value medicinal plant species over the years. The primary threats to medicinal plants are those that affect any kind of biodiversity used by humans. The weakening of customary laws, which have regulated the use of natural resources, are among the causes of threatening the medicinal plant species.

These customary laws have often proved to be easily diluted by modern socio-economic forces. There are many other potential causes of rarity in medicinal plant species, such as habitat specificity, narrow range of distribution, land use disturbances, introduction of non-natives, habitat alteration, climatic changes, heavy livestock grazing, explosion of human population, fragmentation and degradation of population, population bottleneck, and genetic drift. Additionally, natural enemies (*i.e.*, pathogens, herbivores, and seed predators) could substantially limit the abundance of rare medicinal plant species in any given area.

In addition to the consumption of medicinal plants by animals, there are physical ailments in humans, which are cured by different species of the same genera. For example, the malarial fever is treated by many species of Swertia (*e.g.* Swertia chiraiyta, S. angustifolia, and S. cordata). Similarly, different species of Berberis (*e.g.* Berberis aristata, B. asiatica, B. lycium, B. chitria and B. jaeschkeana) are used as a source of berberidine to cure certain eye diseases. Furthermore, different species of the same genera contain different proportions of chemical quantity, and there is a preference over their demand; however, the degree of threat for their exploitation is relatively lower than those species, which do not have alternatives

An estimated 4,000 to 10,000 species of medicinal plants face potential local, national, regional or global extinction, with subsequent serious consequences for livelihoods, economies and health care systems. Although, a few studies exist on the rare and endangered medicinal plant species of the northern India, none of these studies have complete data set for even a single species. In 2003, 71 rare and endangered medicinal plant species have been assessed for the northwest Himalaya during the Conservation Assessment and Management Plan workshop, according to the guidelines of the World Conservation Union. In northern India, Aconitum is the rarest genus with 5 species, followed by Rheum with 4 rare species. Out of the 71 rare medicinal plants, 92% are in active trade; 74% are traded nationally and 35% are traded internationally .

The meager availability of data on the population and quantum of rare species in nature, however, has restricted their categorization to a few species on the basis of herbarium collection and by consultation by a few experts. The present assessments are also questioned for their validity on the assignment of threat categories to the species, including the number of taxa in danger for specific area.

The problems in assessing the species is increased in the mountainous region, especially high altitude areas because of tough and inaccessibility of the terrain, inhospitable climatic conditions, and short life cycle of plants. Most of the available data have been collected from the easily accessible areas in these mountains.

Indigenous communities and commercial herb gatherers also raid these same areas for collection of medicinal plants. Therefore, the estimated population density of categorized rare medicinal plants is not precise because it differs the areas that never and hardly undergone any collection of such rare medicinal plant species.

Cultivation of Medicinal Plants

Information on the propagation of medicinal plants is available for less than 10% and agro-technology is available only for 1% of the total known plants globally. This trend shows that developing agro-technology should be one of the thrust areas for research. Furthermore, in order to meet the escalating demand of medicinal plants, farming of these plant species is imperative. Apart from meeting the present demand, farming may conserve the wild genetic diversity of medicinal plants. Farming permits the production of uniform material, from which standardized products can be consistently obtained. Cultivation also permits better species identification, improved quality control, and increased prospects for genetic improvements.

Selection of planting material for large-scale farming is also an important task. The planting material therefore should be of good quality, rich in active ingredients, pest- and disease-resistant and environmental tolerant. For the large scale farming, one has to find out whether monoculture is the right way to cultivate all medicinal plants or one has to promote polyculture model for better production of medicinal plants.

Studies conducted on the agro-forestry of medicinal plants elsewhere suggest that since many medicinal plant species prefer to grow under forest cover, agroforestry offers a convenient strategy for their cultivation as well as conservation through: (1) integrating shade tolerant medicinal plants as lower strata species in multistrata system, (2) cultivating short cycle medicinal plants as intercrops in existing stands of tree crops, (3) growing medicinal tree as shade providers and boundary markers, and 4) inter-planting medicinal plants with food crops. Notwithstanding, it is understood that the cultivation of medicinal plants is not an easy task as the history of medicinal plants farming reflects.

Many farmers in trans-Himalayan region of northern India have replaced the medicinal plants farming with common crops [*i.e.*, peas (Pisum sativum), potatos (Solanum tuberosum) and hops (Humulus lupulus)] due to the lengthy cultivation cycle of medicinal plants like Saussurea costus. The cost of many medicinal plants in northern India is lower than many seasonal vegetables, which is a cause of scanty farming of medicinal plants.

Attempts are being made by different organizations to cultivate various medicinal plant species, including rare and endangered categories. Agro-technology for about 20 species of rare and endangered medicinal plants of the northern India has been developed by different organizations. However, the per hectare cost of cultivation, total annual production and cost benefit ratio fluctuate with different medicinal plant species. Out of 10 selected rare and endangered medicinal plant species, Rheum emodi was calculated as a most beneficial cash crop of the medicinal plant in terms of net income generation in northern India.

At present, however, the farming of most of the medicinal plant species is being operated on a small scale and is restricted to a few hectares of land in various states of northern India. There is an uncertainty of obtaining the necessary permits from government agencies for cultivation of medicinal plants. Additionally, many farmers are unaware about the agency responsible for issuing permits. If the farmers are not granted permits needed to cultivate, they are forced to sell their products on the illegal market, which exposes them to action by government agencies and the exploitation by middlemen.

Bio-prospecting and Bio-piracy

The former remote green forests have now become part of a dynamic, profit-seeking economy and demanding pluralistic politics worldwide. Reducing the pressure on various forest products, especially on the medicinal plants, is therefore a tough challenge both for policy makers and for economists. Medicinal plants are the local heritage with global importance.

The Convention on Biological Diversity at Rio had agreed on a framework that would help the biodiversity to be utilized in a prudent and controlled way. Bio-prospecting, at present, occurs in an environment of suspicions and growing tensions between the bio-piracy and rights of sharing benefits between the developing and developed countries. Most of the issues relating to the protection of the legal status for indigenous knowledge and compensation of the indigenous herbal practitioners for that knowledge are extremely complicated. There are arguments for the present state of compensation or benefit sharing under the intellectual property rights, which is being considered a new legal form of bio-piracy by one group, whereas other groups argue that the intellectual property right is a legal tool to protect the rights of knowledge holders.

Different ways and systems for awarding patents on the medicinal plants in India, United States, Europe, Canada and other countries have widened the confusion. In many countries, the plants and inventions directed to the plants and the plant products (*i.e.*, seeds, flowers, gums, and resins) are not eligible for filing a patent. In United States, however, any living organism derived by human invention, such as by breeding or by laboratory-based manipulation, can be filed for awarding patent. The Indian Protection of Plant Varieties and Farmers Rights Act of 2001 recognizes the contribution of farmers who actively participate in the breeding programmes. Furthermore, this act contains provisions for benefit sharing whereby local communities are acknowledged as a contributor of plants .

Unfortunately, there is a wide gap between developed and developing nations such as India on patenting the products. For example, out of the 3,125,603 patents filed in 91 countries, only 301,177 or 9.6% are registered in developing countries while the rest is in industrialized countries. Of these, only 0.2% of the total and 2.3% of those registered in developing countries belong to residents. In addition, 97.7% of the total patents filed thus far are in the name of non-residents, who apply solely to control export markets in developing countries.

Developing nations and many scientists who want to exploit medicinal plants demand more specific rules about the recording of nationality of samples and sharing of their benefits between the nations of origin, the inventor, and the commercial sponsors. Some developed nations are not inclined to accept such provisions. These conflicts have frustrated many scientists who believe that natural products remain the most promising source for new drugs. To mitigate such conflicts and gear up to find out new sources for drugs, the representatives of 188 nations at Kuala Lumpur Conference in 2004 agreed to try to build such a framework that would be acceptable to all signatories and thus the proposed framework will be placed for consideration at the next meeting in 2006 going to be held in Brazil.

Strengthening Legalized Market System

Besides government agencies, there are numbers of stake-holders ranging from herb gatherers, local middlemen, urban traders, wholesalers, manufacturers, exporters and herbal healers in the medicinal plants trade sector. The marketing system in medicinal plants sector is largely unregulated and inequitable. The medicinal plant collectors are generally the marginal farmers and labourers. They get cash income to meet their basic requirements for food, health and children education by selling medicinal plants.

They are often unaware about the real market prices of many medicinal plant species. Generally, in medicinal plants sector, there is a top down approach and even the many stake-holders at the bottom are not aware of the rising demand of their product and the availability of its market. In some villages of Chamoli district of Uttaranchal, the farmers had cultivated Kut (Saussurea costus) and Dolu (Rheum emodi) but they were unable to sell them due to lack of knowledge on the marketing system. Conversely, many medicinal plant species are traded through illegal channels.

The other constraints in the medicinal plants sector are: (1) slow rate of production of many medicinal plants, (2) long gestation period, (3) shortage of suitable cultivation technology, (4) production of small quantity, (5) unscientific harvesting, (6) paucity of research on the high yielding varieties, (7) inefficient processing techniques, (8) fluctuation in demand and supply, (9) poor quality control procedures, (10) scarcity of good manufacturers, (11) poor marketing infrastructure, and (12) poor coordination among different stake-holders. On many occasions, the wild medicinal plants are preferred by manufactures compared to the cultivated ones, as there is a general feeling that wild plant species contain better chemical contents. The variation in chemical contents also depends upon the harvesting seasons of species and different stages of species growth. The medicinal plant sector is largely less documented and inadequately regulated. The economy generated by this sector is therefore, not precise because of the enormous illegal trade. The economic benefits and management cost for wild populations are poorly estimated on several occasions.

Opportunities in Developing the Medicinal Plants Sector

For developing the 'herbal industries', the northern India possesses a rich diversity of medicinal plant species across the various forest types along an altitudinal gradient (as discussed in the use and diversity of medicinal plants). Such a high diversity of medicinal plants would be helpful for further scientific research on exploring their medical efficacy, value addition, and use in curing various old and new diseases. India has already established a reputation as a low-cost manufacturer of high quality generic drugs in the global market. This fact can be used as an important tool for the marketing of herbal products produced in India. It is expected that India's aim to build a golden triangle between traditional medicine, modern medicine, and modern science will be a boon for developing the traditional herbal medicine and the medicinal plants sector.

Existing Policies

In the National Five Year Plans of India, the medicinal plants sector has been identified as an integral part of the Indian System of Medicine and Homeopathy. In 1983, the National Health Policy recognized that the large stock of health manpower in Ayurveda, Siddha, Unani, Homeopathy and Naturopathy had not been adequately utilized; therefore, steps need to be taken to move towards a meaningful integration of the indigenous and modern systems of medicine. The Planning Commission and the National Medicinal Plants Board (NMPB) of the Government of India have prepared a policy document on the promotional and commercial aspects of the medicinal plants sector. In addition, the NMPB has prioritized 32 and Planning Commission has enlisted 24 medicinal plant species for research and development in order to meet the desired aim of the medicinal plant sector. The Biodiversity Act 2002 has framed many rules for sustainable utilization of medicinal plants and to mitigate the chances of bio-piracy.

According to Uttaranchal state action plan, the Forest Department of the state will have to identify two major areas in each Forest Division; namely the conservation area and the developmental area. The conservation areas will be selected based on their rich medicinal plants diversity and marked for in-situ conservation and complete protection in the concerned Forest Division. In the developmental areas, apart from protection of the existing bio-resources, the medicinal plant species of the neighbouring areas will also be introduced and cultivated at a large scale.

The remaining areas in the Forest Division will remain open for sustainable harvesting of the medicinal plant species. A Joint Harvesting Team, composed of medicinal plants experts, Forest Department officials and some selected local people, will be constituted, which will decide the extent of annual harvesting of the desired medicinal plant species. The various policies at national and state level and their subsequent implementation will provide an opportunity in the advancement of medicinal plants sector. This model of conservation and cultivation of the medicinal plants may be useful for generating the raw material for the 'Herbal Industries' as well as for ensuring the conservation of the rare medicinal plants.

Institutional Support

In India, many government and non-government organizations have had the focused attention on improving the medicinal plants sector. Opportunities for funding have been created to assist the person who is willing to work and to build capacity of the medicinal plants sector. According to the mandate of NMPB, the projects may be submitted for funding within two major schemes: viz., a promotional scheme and a commercial scheme. The major thrust areas within the promotional scheme are: (1) survey and inventory of medicinal plants, (2) in-situ conservation and ex-situ cultivation of selected medicinal plants, (3) production of quality planting material, (4) diffusion of knowledge through education and communication, (5) promotion of global and domestic market system, and (6) strengthening research, development and man power. Within the commercial scheme, the major thrust areas are: (i) bulk production of medicinal plants and ensuring supply of quality planting material, (ii) expansion of selected medicinal plants farming areas, (iii) value addition in harvesting, processing and marketing of medicinal plants, and (iv) developing innovative marketing mechanism.

Apart from the two major themes, the role of NMPB is to co-ordinate with the different ministries, departments, organizations, state and union territory Governments in order to develop and strengthen the medicinal plant sector. One of the major roles of NMPB is to make contacts with national and international organizations devoted to similar mandates and goals. A total of 35 State Medicinal Plants Boards have also been created by NMPB for the smooth functioning of the medicinal plants sector.

Approximately 35,000 hectares of land has been selected and brought under cultivation under the supervision of NMPB for the large-scale farming of commercially important medicinal plants. One of the schemes of NMPB is a contractual farming in which any group, institution or person that possesses at least 3 years of experience in medicinal plants sector would be eligible to receive at least 30% financial assistance of the total project cost .

Ten years before establishment of NMPB (during 1992-93 financial years), a single project was launched to study the medicinal plants of the Himalayan region. During past one decade, there has been a considerable expansion in the Himalayan medicinal plants research as it is evident that many projects have been launched exclusively on the medicinal plants during that period. Of the total 4254 projects sanctioned by NMPB over past 5 years, 732 projects have been sanctioned to 11 hill states in northern India. All these projects are expected to strengthen the medicinal plants sector, to bridge the gaps and to meet the challenges in developing the sector. In addition to major funding organizations, the G.B. Pant Institute of

Himalayan Environment and Development has sanctioned projects on the medicinal plants of northern India under the scheme of Ministry of Environment & Forests. The Council of Scientific and Industrial Research is building up a Traditional Knowledge Digital Library, which will contain > 35,000 herbal medical formulations used in Ayurvedic system of medicine .

The National Bank for Agriculture and Rural Development (NABARD) has established a policy with a viewpoint to develop a suitable environment for financial institutions by providing bankable models for some 50 medicinal and aromatic crops with the unit cost and scale of finance at the state level. Additionally, NABARD assists in supporting the capacity building of prospective entrepreneurs through Rural Entrepreneurs Development Programmes by providing 100% refinancing. NABARD has also close linkages with the NMPB and different State Medicinal Plants Boards. Attempts have been made by various organizations at different levels to establish and promote the medicinal plants sector.

Recommendations for Developing the Medicinal Plants Sector

The present worldwide interest in plant-based medicines of Indian origin needs to be harnessed by reframing a clear policy for the promotion of commercial cultivation, research and development, and for the increase in exports of medicinal plants. For the development of the medicinal plant sector, there is a need to develop the coordinated efforts at each stage (*e.g.* research, cultivation, collection, storage, processing, manufacturing and marketing), which would be supported by an appropriate policy framework.

Selection of medicinal plant species for cultivation is an initial important step for the development of the medicinal plants sector. Economic feasibility is the major rationale for a decision to bring medicinal plant species into cultivation. Apart from the priority species selected by the Planning Commission and the NMPB, the rare species banned for collection from the wild should also be taken on a priority basis for cultivation because a majority of such species are very expensive, have high demand and low supply. Cultivation may not be economical if a medicinal plant species is abundant in the wild and easily collected. Therefore, the less abundant species in the wild should be promoted for the large-scale cultivation. Farming of any medicinal plant species should be brought into practice only after the reliable cultivation technology of the concerned species is available. A large variation in climatic and soil conditions in northern India sustain a variety of medicinal plant species, which may be cultivated according to their niche.

For developing the medicinal plants sector, there is a need to: (1) document indigenous uses of medicinal plants, (2) certify raw material for quality control, (3) develop and improve the agro-technology for valuable medicinal plants, (4) officially recognize and protect the customary laws of indigenous people, (5) prepare a clear policy for granting permits for cultivation within stipulated time, (6) conduct regular research and training on better harvesting and processing techniques, (7) investigate various pathological agents infecting medicinal plants, (8) setup a community-based management of medicinal plants farming and marketing, (9) analyze the market policies, (10) monitor and evaluate the status of medicinal plants with the assistance of local communities, (11) conserve the critical habitats of rare medicinal plant species, and (12) share benefits judiciously arising from local people's knowledge on medicinal plants. These attempts may reduce dependency on wild resource base, and generate alternative income opportunities for the rural and underprivileged communities.

The medicinal plants sector can be improved if the agricultural support agencies would come forward to help strengthen the medicinal plants growers, and if research institutions would help the plant growers by improving their basic knowledge about cultivation practices. Awareness and interest of farmers, supportive government policies, assured markets, profitable price levels, access to simple and appropriate agro-techniques, and availability of trained manpower are some of the key factors for successful medicinal plants cultivation. The diffusion of any available scientific knowledge on medicinal plants should be made operational by a network structure of communication. Currently there are number of herbs which are used in curing diseases but are not documented in details due to a lack of communication and relatively low frequency of their uses. The traditional uses of low profile and lesser-known medicinal plants should also be documented to disseminate their therapeutic efficacy by preparing well acceptable medicines and also to reduce the pressure on over-exploited species.

Apart from the more than 9992 licensed pharmacies with 717319 registered practitioners of Ayurveda, Siddha, Unani and Homeopathy in India, there are many unregistered herbal practitioners in India who prepare their own traditional herbal formulations for curing different diseases, and the available herbal formulations should be standardized for their efficacy. Such scientifically prepared medicine will place herbal medicine in a proper perspective and help in getting a broad global market. Some people do try to take advantage through the introduction of less effective medicinal plants in the name of well-established high-value medicinal plants.

Such attempts must be discouraged. To discourage such malpractices, the certification of raw material should be done for quality control by using the modern tools such as thin layer chromatography and high performance thin layer chromatography. In addition, high performance liquid chromatography (HPLC), volumetric analysis, gas chromatography, column chromatography, and gravimetric determinations may be used for standardization and for quality control. Various factors relating to pathological agents (*e.g.* bacteria, virus, fungi and nematodes) and infected medicinal plants should be investigated by identifying the various symptoms of diseases such as mildew, rust, necrosis, spots, blight, rot, wilt, galls, curl and canker to produce the healthy farming of medicinal plants.

On many occasions, the collection of planting material, especially of rare and endangered medicinal plant species from natural habitats for various experimental purposes by researchers, also poses a threat on their natural populations in wild. The researchers must be aware on the germination potential, seedlings and rhizomes survival strategies of the desired species collected from wild for scientific experiments. Researchers must plant a similar number of individuals back in nature after completion of research work on the collected species. There is also a communication problem between researchers and farmers. This communication problem limits a researcher's capability to deal with the farmers' problems. Hence, communication links between researchers, extension services of institutions, and farmers should be strengthened.

The majorities of current research programmes on the medicinal plants conservation are being shifted from ecosystems to species levels. Although there are protected areas across the Himalaya, most of the protected areas have a focused attention on the preservation of faunal diversity except for a few protected areas such as the Valley of Flowers in North West Himalaya and the Tipi Orchid Sanctuary in North East Himalaya. There is not a single protected area focusing on the conservation of medicinal plants.

Thus, there is an urgent need for identification and notification of areas for the conservation of medicinal plants on a priority basis. Most of the documentation and research on indigenous uses of medicinal plants is focused on the human aspect. Animal husbandry is the backbone of economy in a majority of indigenous societies. Maintaining the good health of livestock will benefit these indigenous societies. Since there are many medicinal plant species used in curing the various animal related disorders and diseases, the research work also needs to be done on the uses of medicinal plants for curing livestock diseases.

Being a part of tradition, there are many other social issues attached with medicinal plants sector. The indigenous knowledge on harvesting, storage and usage of medicinal plants built over centuries needs to be taken into account for improving the sector and allocating scare resources among the competing demands. Development of medicinal plants farming, encouragement of traditional herbal use and herbal healers, establishing medicinal plants conservation areas, establishing the Social Capital Trust for herbal healers, establishment of linkages among various stake-holders, etc., are among some of the social issues that need to be honored and addressed properly. The folklore on several medicinal plants and the formulation developed by using them is well recognized in different ethnic communities living in northern India. These folklores should be brought into laboratory for validation.

Medicinal Plants—The Global View

Human beings have been utilizing plants for basic preventive and curative health care since time immemorial. Recent estimates suggest that over 9,000 plants have known medicinal applications in various cultures and countries, and this is without having conducted comprehensive research amongst several indigenous and other communities (Farnsworth and Soejarto 1991).

Medicinal plants are used at the household level by women taking care of their families, at the village level by medicine men or tribal shamans, and by the practitioners of classical traditional systems of medicine such as Ayurveda, Chinese medicine, or the Japanese Kampo system. According to the World Health Organization, over 80% of the world's population, or 4.3 billion people, rely upon such traditional plant-based systems of medicine to provide them with primary health care (Bannerman et. al. 1983).

Allopathic medicine too owes a tremendous debt to medicinal plants: one in four prescriptions filled in a country like the United States are either a synthesized form of or derived from plant materials (Srivastava, et. al. 1995). Even from the earliest trade data available, it is clear that the global market for medicinal plants has always been very large.

According to the International Trade Centre, as far back as 1967, the total value of imports of starting materials of plant origin for the pharmaceutical and cosmetics industry was of the order of USD 52.9 million. From this amount, the total values grew to USD 71.2 million in 1971, and then showed a steady annual growth rate of approximately 5-7% through to the mid-1980s (Atisso 1983).

To give an example of the extent of trade volumes even at that time, according to one report commissioned by the World Wide Fund for Nature, the total import in 1980 of "vegetable materials used in pharmacy" by the European Economic Community was 80,738 tons (Lewington 1992). India was the largest supplier by far, with 10,055 tons of plants and 14 tons of vegetable alkaloids and their derivatives.

However, it is only during the last decade that the real significance of the medicinal plants sector has begun to be realized. Interest in natural materials by the dominant economic powers had waned from the late 1960s to the early 1980s as new possibilities in biotechnology and the synthesization of drugs beckoned. But by the mid-1980s, there was a renewed interest in natural materials and approaches to health care, coupled with a recognition that technology alone could not solve the pressing health care needs of the world's population (Tempesta and King 1994).

This new drive for natural and plant-based medicines made itself felt in the market from the mid-1980s onwards. As table illustrates, growth in the market in various regions is now on average 3 to 4 times the average growth rates of the national economies in the same regions. Some of these phenomenal rates, in some cases nearly 20%, imply that the market is now doubling in size every 4-5 years.

The participation of various companies in the market also attests to its new strength and importance. By 1990, some 223 major companies worldwide (of which about half were in the United States) were reportedly screening plants for new leads; the figure had been zero in 1980 (Aryal 1993).

Also in 1990, more than 2000 companies in Europe alone were marketing herbal medicinals, with 30% having a turnover in excess of $20 million- expenditure in the United States on "unconventional, alternative, or unorthodox" therapies reached $13.7 billion dollars during the same year (Tewari 1996). The so-called "nutraceuticals" sector—consisting of herbal medicines which are dubbed food or dietary supplements in order to pass FDA criteria more easily—is now estimated to be valued at USD 27 billion (Anon 1995).

Natural Medicines Market: Regional Growth Rates 1991-98 (in %)

Region	*1991-92*	*1993-98*
EU	5	8
Rest of Europe	8	12
SE Asia	12	12
Japan	15	15
South Asia	15	15

(1994) Source: Grunwald

The use of such alternative medicines has become increasingly popular in the developed world. For example, 1 in 3 Americans have at some time used unconventional medical therapies according to a national telephone survey published in the New England Journal of Medicine in 1993. In another survey conducted in 1994, it was found that 60% of doctors had at some time referred patients to practitioners of alternative medicine.

In response to the overwhelming interest in alternative therapies, many of the prestigious allopathic medical institutions have also recognized their importance: an example is the National Institute of Health which created the Office of Alternative Medicine in 1991 to provide the public with information on alternative treatments and to assess those therapies which have proven successful. (Kolata 1996).

According to one account, in 1992 significant amounts of at least 74 species of medicinal plants were being commercially traded in the global market (Handa 1992). In addition to these major species, hundreds of others are bought and sold in lesser quantities across national boundaries, sometimes illegally.

A comparison of the volumes of traded materials with those of the previous decade also provides dramatic evidence of the market's growth. During the last 3 years, approximately 40,000 tons of plant drug materials (valued at DM 160 million) were imported into Germany, annually (Lange 1996), implying that one country's imports in the mid 1990s equalled half the number of plants imported by the entire continent in the mid 1980s.

Considering the Role for India

The global context briefly sketched above suggests several tremendous opportunities for India, a country unrivaled in terms of diversity of medical systems and practices, in addition to being a major storehouse of biological diversity, with 2 of the 14 megabiodiversity areas of the world located within its borders. The global market would appear to be more receptive than ever to the mounting of a concentrated Indian effort at supplying it with medical materials and know-how.

Such an effort would also appear to be increasingly remunerative for the country. India is of course already an active participant in the global medicinal plants market having been for some time the world's largest supplier of raw materials (though an insignificant supplier of finished products) (Patnaik 1994). Of the 74 species accounted for in one of the studies mentioned above, India was known to be exporting 22 and importing 8 (Handa 1992), while the German study quoted earlier, which is now underway, has found India to be Germany's largest trading partner by far (Lange 1996). Moreover, medicinal plants are one of the most important components of the non-wood forest products sector which supplies over 80% of India's net forest annual export earnings (FAO 1995, Jain 1996).

Despite these promising indications, however, it is unclear whether India is truly exploiting her comparative advantage in the medicinal plants sector and tapping the full potential of an expanding consumer base. In addition, several concerns arise in relation to the current consequences of participation in the market, with regard to the sustainability and equitability of prevailing practices in the sector.

Although only micro-studies are currently available in this regard, most of these indicate that current practices are both unsustainable, as they rapidly deplete the natural supplies of the country's plant base, and inequitable, perpetuating impoverishment for those charged with stewarding and harvesting the resource, while a few profit in dramatic disproportion to their inputs. Negative impacts on local primary health care, as plants become diverted to national and international markets, have also been cited in some cases. To add to all of these negative aspects, the market in India has been shown to be highly inefficient and imperfect.

The need of the hour, then, is to replan India's participation in the expanding global market, in light of the interests of all the stake-holders who are affected and who play a role in this sector. There is a need to collate all the available information regarding medicinal plants development in the country in order to obtain a comprehensive overview which will provide the necessary insight for coordinated and effective action. Such an overview could form the basis of a renewed development of India's medicinal plants sector, and a strategic exploitation of her comparative advantage in the global market on a sustainable and equitable basis.

Origins and Objectives of the Review

It was with the intention of providing such a comprehensive overview that the International Development Research Centre and the World Bank's Department of Agriculture and Natural Resources commissioned the authors to conduct a state-of-the-art review of the medicinal plants sector in India.

Medicinal plants, of course, do not presently constitute a sector as typically defined in international development discourse; generally they have been defined as a forestry sub-sector, or less often, as a sub-sector in health care. However, this review takes up medicinal plants as an independent sector for two reasons: (1) to emphasize that none of the various 'homes' to which medicinal plants have been assigned provide a sufficient base of expertise for their sustainable and equitable development; and (2) to provide an organizational framework for the community of researchers and stake-holders, to whom this paper will be circulated, to think through this area of common interest and move forward together.

This review then is a mapping exercise, which tries to identify the who, what, how, where, why and when of medicinal plants development in India, in order to supply a comprehensive understanding and overall picture to researchers, NGOs, health care workers, private companies, conservation and development agencies, policy makers and other interested stake-holders. It is intended to provide a framework and knowledge base, and an initial way forward, for those interested in seeing India exploit her comparative advantage in the global market, both sustainably and equitably.

Limits and Constraints Faced

There is no dearth of interest in medicinal plants amongst the Indian research community. As a single example, the IDRC Medicinal Plants Network, a South-Asia focused initiative operating from New Delhi, already maintains an active database of over 900 Indian researchers and development specialists working on medicinal plants projects after only one year of active compilation. When a call for proposals in the field was issued, over 250 responses were received within the subscribed period, a tremendous number considering that the grants were of the magnitude of only USD 15,000.

Unfortunately, however, this interest has not resulted in the development of a strong and high-quality knowledge base for the sector. Instead, one finds in a review such as this one several instances where information is either unobtainable or unreliable. Several factors contribute to this situation.

The most important among these is the highly secretive and complex nature of the trade in raw materials. Most experts consulted agreed that the largest part of the trade occurs in the informal sector, and is absent from official statistics and trade catalogues. As previous authors have also found (see Lewington 1993), nearly everyone involved in the medicinal plants trade is very hesitant to divulge information which is essential to a complete understanding—such as prices, supply sources, points of transformation, and transport routes. As a result, despite assiduous efforts, we still cannot claim to have a complete picture of the trade scenario, and have most likely erred in the direction of conservatively estimating the volumes of materials under trade.

Information available regarding the formal sector is also limited. Most data is available only in aggregate form, such as numbers of species being exported or overall value of the trade to India. These statistics unfortunately supply little information about how the market actually works, and may even obscure such vital information to policy makers such as seasonal fluctuations and the like. In addition, in most cases, no explanations are given for how the aggregations were calculated or verified (*i.e.* dry weights or fresh weights; exchange values in effect; self-reporting by companies or based on registration with governments, etc.). The lack of methodological explanation makes it virtually impossible to compare and synthesize related sets of information; or to understand why two sets of statistics, purporting to cover the same phenomena over the same time period, give differing results.

Moreover, these statistics rely exclusively on market price as an indicator of value, a narrow approach which neglects environmental, cultural, personal, and long-term methods of assigning value. The social context of the market which is extremely important in the medicinal plants sector, involving as it does, a complex market spread across time and space, is there by lost.

This constraint is related to a general lack of strategic focus in the bulk of current socio-economic research on medicinal plants in India. The largest group of scientists currently working with medicinal plants appears to be those in the natural sciences—including botanists, taxonomists, and chemists; and the applied sciences such as biotechnology and health care. In most instances where economic or social analysis has been undertaken, it has been by these same scientists, the majority of whom are untrained and unqualified to conduct such research. While laudable as an attempt to bridge the disciplinary barrier, this has unfortunately also resulted in a generally lower quality of socio-economic analysis related to medicinal plants as against other resources, with analysis tending to oversimplify complex market and policy realities such as the frequently suggested solution: cut out the middleman. In addition, there is a regrettable absence of any 'research community' or peer group working on socio-economic and policy aspects of medicinal plants, such as that which exists with regard to agro-technology, biotechnology, and the like, which would assist in defining higher standards of quality.

Methodology

The consequences of the absence of an extensive knowledge base is that in many places there remain gaps which need to be filled; where these occur, the study takes note of them. However, these have not been so numerous as to make it impossible to give a reasonable picture of the sector. In the absence of the usual sources of information for commodity studies, this review utilizes a hybrid approach following in part the model articulated by Arnold (1994).

The review attempts to understand the market by means of the 'official' sources available regarding the macro-level trade, as well as the few well-documented case studies of the micro-level situation, supplemented by interviews and discussions with experts in the field who are participants in the IDRC Medicinal Plants Network. Where common trends and tendencies appear, they are highlighted; and where gaps remain, they are acknowledged. In this way, the review serves as a stock-taking not only of the development scenario, but of the research scenario as well.

The review is structured to follow the medicinal plants from their origins in forests and on farms through to their application in formulations or as unprocessed materials. For this purpose, we have identified five major stages which medicinal plants may pass through on their way from collection to use.

Different people and plants are engaged at each stage, and the review attempts to provide information on not only on the volumes and numbers of people involved; but also to understand which ones are involved, why they are involved, how and to what extent they are involved, and when they are involved. It also tries to understand and describe how changes at different points have affected the participation of people and plants at the same or other points. Such factors are of crucial importance in considering development initiatives for the sector.

Industry Roles in Medicinal Plant Conservation

This is the story of one company's efforts to source its herbal ingredients from sustainable sources, according to its own account. Pukka Herbs, founded in the UK in 1999, imports plant materials from India and Sri Lanka for the manufacture of ayurvedic preparations. In an interview with Alan Hamilton of Plantlife International, Sebastian Pole, co-founder of Pukka Herbs, emphasised his company's interest in providing high quality health-giving products. Sebastian believes that organic production can be a key to such quality assurance. As with ecological sustainability, verification of organic status requires traceability back to the source areas of the plants, so that Pukka Herbs has a prima-facie motivation to establish traceability.

Pukka Herbs does not buy raw plant materials directly from individual farmers or collectors (which would be a hard task for all but the smallest manufacturers), but does have close relationships with producer companies that work closely with farmers. Pukka does try to restrain the length of its supply chains (which tend to be extensive in the herbal business). Long supply chains, with many intermediate traders between producers and manufacturers, compound the difficulties of tracing the movements of plant materials. They make it difficult for manufacturers to verify that adequate 'production quality' has been achieved for any of the quality categories in which they might be interested - ecological sustainability, product quality (such as organic) and fair trade.

A maximum of three trade links separates Pukka Herbs from the producers of the medicinal plants and usually only two. Pukka purchases plant materials from exporting companies in India and Sri Lanka, that either buy these materials directly from the producers or else buy them from intermediate companies that themselves are directly connected.

Exporting Company—Pukka Herbs

Pukka's ability to achieve traceability for its raw materials, as well as required standards of organic production, has been recognised by the Soil Association, with Pukka's products certified as organic to EU and US standards (the latter under the National Organic Programme). Field certification was by the certifiers SKAL and ECOCERT, their certification being passed on to the Soil Association through recognition of standards' equivalence. Certification was to the normal organic standard of the Soil Association (used mainly for cultivated plants) and not to according to its Organic Wild Crafting Standard, which has more stringent sustainability requirements relating specifically to wild plants.

Principles of 'Production Quality' and their Sharing

Pukka's relationships with a few exporting companies in India and Sri Lanka are central to its business. These exporters are reported by Pukka Herbs to be ecologically and ethically minded agricultural companies that purchase crops from farmers, as well as providing them with training, advice, seeds and fair-trade relationships. Pukka's trading partners were not involved in some of the more specialised Ayurvedic medicinal plants prior to their relationships with Pukka.

Pukka Herbs is committed through its business principles to high quality in three aspects of production: high quality ingredients from the medicinal perspective, ecological sustainability and fair trade. As regards sustainability, Pukka Herbs has its own working document on standards and guidelines to guide its efforts to achieving sustainable harvest. This document is based closely on the standards of the Soil Association, covering both cultivated and wild plants. Special emphasis is placed on the need for management systems for wild plants to be adaptive, allowing rapid and appropriate response to changing circumstances.

The social agenda of Pukka Herbs aims to enhance the livelihoods of the producers of the medicinal plants through enhancing their autonomy. Specific objectives are to develop long-term relationships with the producers (including for the promotion of sustainable production practices and long-term planning), the payment of premium prices that include the cost of sustainable production, the provision of technical assistance and advice, the encouragement or strengthening of community groups for self-empowerment, and the promotion of local markets for organic production (to spread the risks to the producers, so that they are not uniquely bound to Pukka Herbs for market access).

Pukka's business principles must be shared by its business partners in India and Sri Lanka, if they are to be carried into effect. It is these business partners that can give field reality to Pukka's own objectives, which, in the sustainability arena, include the establishment of systems of sustainable harvesting for wild plants, the training of farmers in organic agriculture and assistance for the establishment of nurseries (whether to produce seedlings for field crops or for enrichment planting in the wild).

Pukka Herbs has developed memoranda of understanding (MOU) with its business partners regarding intentions, aspirations and operating standards, covering:

- Organic farming standards
- Commitment to fair trade
- Medicinal plant quality
- Processing standards
- Attainment of Good Agricultural Practice (GAP) and Good Manufacturing Practice (GMP).

Pukka Herbs undertakes an annual exercise in relationship building, technical auditing and quality inspection at randomly selected growing and processing areas to ensure that the terms of the MOU are being met. Relationships are being built 'inclusively', recognising that current practices are not perfect, but rather 'work-in-progress'. The company reports that, with a willingness to learn and a spirit of co-operation, steady progress is proving possible, year-by-year.

The Forest Gardens

Most of the plant materials purchased by Pukka Herbs are actually derived from field crops, rather than wild plants. Of course, there are benefits for plant conservation from organic agriculture, but the parts of Pukka's business most strongly relevant to wider plant conservation are two cases of harvesting wild or semi-wild plants in Sri Lanka. One of these involves the production of medicinal plants in 'forest gardens' and the other the collection of medicinal plants from natural habitats. The exceptional plant conservation interests here are the possibilities of conserving natural populations of plants with their genetic diversity and ecological connections, and opportunities to provide incentives for the conservation of natural or semi-natural habitats containing a diversity of plants.

The forest (or home) gardens of Sri Lanka are famous for their plant diversity, with a total of more than 400, mostly indigenous, species of woody plants recorded. These gardens are tended patches of vegetation of intermediate status between fully wild and fully domesticated. Found in all climatic parts of the island - from the wet rainforest regions of the southwest and centre to the drier wooded savannas of the north and east- the forest gardens of Sri Lanka are economically important to the nation, being the source of 41 per cent of its saw-logs and 26 per cent of its biofuel (Ariyadasa 2002; FSMP 1995). They contain a large number of medicinal plants, including the scrambler Asparagus racemosus, the small shrub Munronia pinnata, the large climbers Coscinum fenestratum and Tinospora cordifolia, and the trees Strychnos nux-vomica and Syzygium cumini.

For the purposes of judging ecological sustainability, a choice must be made for the forest gardens as whether to regard them as cultivated or wild. Sustainability can be judged very differently in the two cases. As typically defined, sustainable agriculture refers to a quite different set of required criteria to sustainability for a wild plant resource. Sustainable agriculture primarily requires maintenance of the basic quality of the land, particularly as regards the quality of the soil, and there is no special need for continuing production of any particular crop in a particular field. In contrast, sustainability with reference to a wild plant resource typically requires that the resource re-grows - most stringently defined as reforming at a rate at least as fast as its rate of extraction.

For the purposes of resource management (as opposed to certification requirements), Pukka Herbs decided to regard the forest gardens as wild rather than cultivated (an excellent decision from the wider plant conservation perspective). There then ensued questions about how to ensure that the management and harvesting of medicinal plants in these gardens conformed to standards required for sustainability.

Developing Management Systems for the Forest Gardens

Garden ownership, allowable off-take and enrichment planting were among matters that required addressing to establish satisfactory systems of garden management for sustainability.

On ownership, it is widely recognised that a key requirement for proper management of a natural resource is security of rights over its use. For example, the Organic Wild Crafting Standard of the Soil Association requires the designation of a responsible manager for each production area. When Pukka Herbs turned its attention to the forest gardens, it discovered that many were not legally registered, creating an obstacle for certification and possibly also for good management.

A lack of legal title for land or plant resources is a common condition in many developing countries and does not necessarily imply a lack of proper management. Customary rules that are publicly respected can also convey the necessary degree of recognised authority. However, in this case, Pukka Herbs, in association with a producing partner (Lanka Organics), considered it necessary to devote considerable effort to getting the land registered, so that the farmers then legally owned the land and their produce could be certified as organic.

The approach taken to setting levels of off-take for the forest gardens was to request officers from the Forest Department to set annual quotas for each species to be harvested, based on discussions with the producer companies and the farmers, and judgements of the levels at which they could be sustainably harvested in particular gardens. These estimates were rule-of-thumb assessments, based on fairly casual observations of the abundance of the species and general knowledge of their ecologies.

No precise measurements were made of the amounts of the species present or of their rates of regeneration or re-growth. In view of the many uncertainties, the levels of allowable off-take were set conservatively, following the precautionary principle. The Forest Department undertakes annual inspections to verify adherence to the set harvesting levels.

The owners of the forest gardens were encouraged to establish small nurseries of some valuable medicinal plants to produce seedlings for enrichment planting. Criteria for species selection included appropriateness for growing in particular climatic regions, saleability and price. Only local and indigenous species were used, examples including Phyllanthus emblica, Piper longum and Tinospora cordifolia.

Harvesting Medicinal Plants from Natural Habitats

The other example of special relevance for wider plant conservation is also in Sri Lanka and concerns the harvesting of medicinal plants in an area of natural forest. The site, near the town of Bibile in the 'intermediate' climatic zone of Sri Lanka, had earlier been chosen as one of five representative Medicinal Plant Conservation Areas (MPCA) in Sri Lanka by a project of the World Conservation Union (IUCN).

The MPCA at Bibile consists of a core forested area and a surrounding zone with farms. During its period of involvement, the IUCN project started to develop systems of sustainable harvesting for medicinal plants in buffer zones of the forest, as well as inaugurating a medicinal plant demonstration garden and involving around 50 local farmers in medicinal plant production.

However, linkages to the market were poor and, as its project came to an end, IUCN requested Lanka Organics in partnership with Pukka Herbs to see whether it could assist the initiatives that it had started to continue and be developed. As a consequence, Lanka Organics, a local business associate of Pukka, has helped some local farmers to achieve certified organic production of medicinal plants and assisted in the development of sustainable harvesting systems for a few species of wild medicinal trees.

The species selected for sustainable wild production are all plants in which it is the fruits that are required by the medicinal trade, making over-harvesting less of a worry than it would be, for example, if it was roots that were needed. They include Phyllanthus emblica, Terminalia cheluba and T. bellirica.

Possible Future Steps

This case study raises questions about how best to develop practical management and harvest guidelines for each species of medicinal plant harvested from natural vegetation at a particular location. Detailed information on the abundance, regeneration and re-growth rates of harvested species has either been unavailable or not of practical use, either in the case of the forest gardens or at Bibile. Rather, the approach used has been to set conservative limits to the types or amounts of products allowed for harvest, based on rule-of-thumb estimates of species abundance and recovery rates, and the likely damage likely to be incurred to the plants through collection. Species- and site-specific collection guidelines may be further developed.

A related issue is about how far quantitative rigour is required or possible for the certification of wild-collected medicinal plants as sustainable. In the present case, organic certification was achieved without the need for a high degree of quantitative rigour in resource assessment or monitoring. Conservation organisations have recently been giving increased thought to certification schemes for sustainability, sometimes requiring many measurements and observations on the status of medicinal species and their habitats to achieve certification.

On the other hand, the herbal and botanical sectors are beset with increasing amounts of regulations, compliance with which can be especially difficult for smaller companies, and there are also the challenges of finding finance and expertise required for sophisticated schemes. The challenge of developing workable systems for certifying sustainable wild collection remains.

Medicinal Plants

Traditional medicines are used by about 60 per cent of the world's population. These are not only used for primary health care not just in rural areas in developing countries, but also in developed countries as well where modern medicines are predominantly used. While the traditional medicines are derived from medicinal plants, minerals, and organic matter, the herbal drugs are prepared from medicinal plants only.

Use of plants as a source of medicine has been inherited and is an important component of the health care system in India. In the Indian systems of medicine, most practitioners formulate and dispense their own recipes, hence this requires proper documentation and research.

In western world also, the use of herbal medicines is steadily growing with approximately 40 per cent of population reporting use of herb to treat medical illnesses within the past year. Public, academic and government interest in traditional medicines is growing exponentially due to the increased incidence of the adverse drug reactions and economic burden of the modern system of medicine.

There are about 45,000 plant species in India, with concentrated hotspots in the region of Eastern Himalayas, Western Ghats and Andaman & Nicobar Island. The officially documented plants with medicinal potential are 3000 but traditional practitioners use more than 6000. India is the largest producer of medicinal herbs and is appropriately called the botanical garden of the world.

There are currently about 250 000 registered medical practitioners of the Ayurvedic system (total for all traditional systems: approximately 291 000), as compared to about 700,000 of the modern medicine system. In rural India, 70 per cent of the population is dependent on the traditional system of medicine, the Ayurveda.

Bibliography

Adams H.: *Hot Pepper Improvement*, St. Michael, CARDI, 1997.

Agarwal P. K.: *Improvement of Citrus*, New Delhi, Malhotra Publishing House, 1993.

Alexander M. P. and Ganeshan S.: *Pollen Storage*, New Delhi, Malhotra Publishing House, 1993.

Andrews J.: *The Domesticated Capsicums*, University of Texas Press. 1995.

Andrews L.: *Citrus Production - Orange*, St. Augustine, Trinidad and Tobago, 1990

————: *Production of Minor Crops Sapodilla, Tamarind, Guava and Genip*, Port of Spain, Trinidad and Tobago, 1996.

Arguello D. S.: *Production, Post-harvest Management and Exportation of Tropical Fruits in Costa Rica*, Wageningen, Technical Centre for Agricultural and Rural Cooperation, 1992.

Ashworth S.: *Seed to Seed*, Decorah, Seed Savers Publications, 1991.

Barbeau G.: *Tropical Fruits in Nicaragua*, Managua, Nicaragua Ministerio de Desarrollo Agropecuario, Agraria, 1990.

Batlle I. and Tous J.: *Carob Tree (Ceratonia siliqua L.)*. Rome, International Plant Genetic Resources Institute, 1997.

Berger, P.L.: *Pyramids of Sacrifice: Political Ethics and Social Change*, New York, Basic Books, 1974.

————: *Pyramids of Sacrifice: Political Ethics and Social Change*, New York, Basic Books, 1974.

Brooks, D.: *Water: Local-Level Management*, Ottawa, International Development Research Centre, 2002.

Bunnik J. S. C.: *Fresh Fruits and Vegetable: a Survey on the Netherlands and other Major Markets in the European*

Community, Netherlands, Centre for the Promotion of Imports from Developing Countries, 1990.

Burton W.G.: *The Potato*, Holland, H. Veenman & Zonen N.V., 1966.

Cao Van P.: *An Integrated Approach for the Production and Processing of Minor Fruits in Martinique (FWI)*, Port of Spain, Trinidad and Tobago, 1996.

Cardona M. J. G., Carvajal S. L. B., Salinas D. G. C. and Isaza R. G. B. : *Proceedings of the International Seminar on Plantain Production, Quindio, Colombia,* Quindio, Corporation Colombiana de Investigation Agropecuaria, 1998.

Chadha K. L. and Pareek O. P.: *Advances in Horticulture: Fruit Crops,* New Delhi, Malhotra Publishing House, 1993.

Chambers, R.: *Rural Development: Putting the Last First*, London, Longman, 1983.

Collymore L.: *Fruit Production in Barbados*, Port of Spain, Trinidad and Tobago, 1996.

Coste R.: *Coffee: the Plant and the Product*, London, MacMillan, 1992.

Crucefix D.: *Avocado Variety Selection for Export Development,* Roseau, CARDI, 1996.

Cull Brian & Lindsay Pax: *Fruit Growing in Warm Climates for Commercial Growers & Home Gardeners*, Australia, Reed Books, 1995.

Currah L. and Proctor F. J.: *Onions in Tropical Regions*, Kent, Natural Resources Institute, 1990.

Daniells J.: *Illustrated Guide to the Identification of Banana varieties in the South Pacific*, Canberra, ACIAR, 1995.

Degras L.: *Yam: a Tropical Root Crop*, Wageningen, CTA/ MacMillan, 1993.

Dhatt A. S. and Singh Z.: *Propagation and Rootstocks of Citrus*, New Delhi, Malhotra Publishers, 1993.

Diederichsen A.: *Coriander (Coriandrum sativum L.)*. Rome, International Plant Genetic Resources Institute, 1996.

Doijode S. D.: *Seed Germination in Fruits*, New Delhi, Malhotra Publishers, 1993.

Dudley, E.: *The Critical Villager: Beyond Community Participation*, London, Routledge, 1993.

Featherly H. I.: *Taxonomic Terminology of the Higher Plants*, USA, Iowa State College Press, 1954.

Ferentinos L.: *Proceeding of the Sustainable Taro Culture for the Pacific Conference*, Honolulu, HITAHR, 1993.

Forde S: *Proceedings of CARDI / CTA Workshop on Marketability of Caribbean Minor Fruits*, Port of Spain, Trinidad and Tobago, 1996.

Georges, S.: *The Debt Boomerang: How Third World Debt Harms Us All*, Boulder, Westview Press, 1992.

Glowinski Louis: *The Complete Book of Fruit Growing in Australia*, Australia, Lothian Publishing Company Pty. Ltd., 1991.

Godden G.: *Growing Citrus Trees*, Australia, Lothian Publishing Company Pvt. Ltd., 1988.

Gowen S.: *Banana and Plantains*, London, Chapman Hall, 1996.

Green S.K. and Kim J. S.: *Sources of Resistance to Viruses of Pepper (Capsicum spp.): a Catalogue*, Taipei, AVRDC, 1994.

Gunjate R. T. and Tawde A. B.: *Propagation and Rootstocks of Mango*, New Delhi, Malhotra, 1993.

Hartley W.: *A Checklist of Economic Plants in Australia*, Melbourne, C.S.I.R.O., 1979.

Harwood, R. R.: *Marshalling Technology for Development: Proceedings of a Symposium*, Washington, DC, National Academy Press, 1995.

Herklots G. A. C.: *Vegetables in South East Asia*, London, George Allen & Unwin Ltd., 1972.

Hessayon D. G. Dr.: *The Vegetable Expert*, England, PBI, Publications, 1985.

Huaman Z.: *Descriptors for Sweet Potato*, Rome, International Board for Plant Genetic Resources, 1991.

Hurst Jacqui & Rutherford Lyn.: *A Gourmet's Book of Mushrooms & Truffles*, Sydney, Golden Press Pvt. Ltd., 1991.

Jacquat Christiane: *Plants from the Markets of Thailand*, Bangkok, Duang Kamol, 1990.

Jeffers P.: *Evaluation of Four Onion Varieties in Montserrat*, Plymouth, CARDI, 1992.

Kenridge K. C. and Hardy B.: *Biology and Agronomy of Forage Arachis*, Cali, International Centre for Tropical Agriculture, 1994.

Kroll R.: *Cut Flowers*, Wageningen, CTA, 1995.

Kunelius T.: *Annual Ryegrasses in Atlantic Canada*, Ottawa, Agriculture Canada, 1991.

Lofgren, H., Richards, A.: *Food Security, Poverty, and Economic Policy in the Middle East and North Africa*, Washington, DC, International Food Policy Research Institute, 2003.

Mabberley D. J.: *The Plant-Book : a Portable Dictionary of the Vascular Plants*, Cambridge, Cambridge University Press, 1997.

Madulid Domingo A.: *A Pictorial Cyclopedia of Philippine Ornamental Plants*, Philippines, Makati Metro Manila, 1995.

Malins A.: *Postharvest Handling of Pineapple and Mango*, Port of Spain, Trinidad and Tobago, 1992.

Mannetje, L. T. & Jones, R. M.: *Plant Resources of South-East Asia,* Wageningen, Pudoc Scientific Publishers, 1992.

Matsuoka H.: *Cultivation of Panicum Genetic Resources for Evaluation of Characteristics*, Tokyo, JICA, 1997.

Mc Donald F.: *Plant Tissue Culture Manual for Yam, Cassava, Sweet Potato, Dasheen (taro) and Tannia (cocoyam)*, Roseau, Dominica and Cave Hill, 1993.

Mellor, J. W.: *The New Economics of Growth*, Ithaca, Cornell University Press, 1976.

Miller William: *Dictionary of English Plant Names*, London, John Murray, 1884.

Mitra S.: *Postharvest Physiology and Storage of Tropical and Subtropical Fruits*, Oxon, CABI, 1997.

Morris M. L. : *Maize Seed Industries in Developing Countries*, Colorado, Lynne Rienner, 1998.

Morton Julia F.: *Fruits of Warm Climates*, Miami, Julia F. Morton Publisher, 1987.

Murali T. P. and Duncan E. J.: *In Vitro Propagation of Banana through Aseptic Manipulation of Male Inflorescences*, Port of Spain, NIHERST, 1990.

Nabhan G. P.: *Wild Phaseolus Ecogeography in the Sierra Madre Occidental, Mexico: Areographic Techniques for Targeting and Conserving Species Diversity*, Rome, International Board for Plant Genetic Resources, 1990.

Nijdam J. & De Jong A.: *Elsevier's Dictionary of Horticulture in Nine Languages*, Elsevier Scientific Publishing Co. Amsterdam; New York.

Oka H. I.: *Origin of Cultivated Rice*, Elsevier, Japan Scientific Societies Press, 1988.

Oldham P.: *Cost of Production of Major Tree Crops in Dominica*, Roseau, Ministry of Agriculture, 1991.

Ou Yang Jue Ya: *Comparative Study of Mandarin and Cantonese*, Beijing, China Social Sciences Publishing House, 1993.

Percival John: *The Wheat Plant - A Monograph*, London, Duckworth & Co., 1921.

Pilgrim R.: *Post Harvest Handling of Minor Exotics*, St. George's, Grenada, 1996.

Ragone D.: *Breadfruit: Artocarpus Altilis (Parkinson) Fosberg*, Rome, International Plant Genetic Resources Institute, 1997.

Rehm Sigmund: *Multilingual Dictionary of Agronomic Plants*, Boston, Kluwer Academic Publishers, 1994.

Roy S. K.: *Research on Multipurpose Tree Species in Asia: In Vitro Clonal Propagation of Artocarpus Heterophyllus*, Bangkok, Winrock International Institute for Agricultural Development, 1991.

Singh H. P. and Chadha K. L.: *Genetic Resources of Citrus*, New Delhi, Malhotra Publishing House, 1993.

Sinha G. C., Reddy Y. T. N. and Singh G.: *Propagation and Rootstocks in Guava*, New Delhi, Malhotra Publishers, 1993.

Sperling L. and Berkowitz P. *Partners in selection: bean breeders and women bean experts in Rwanda*. Washington, USA: CGIAR, 1994.

Sreekumar V., Indrasenan G and Mammen G.: *Studies of the Quantitative and Qualitative Attributes of Ginger Cultivars*, Calicut, Kasaragod, 1990.

Stover R. H. and Simmonds N. W.: *Bananas*, United Kingdom: Longman Scientific and Technical, 1991.

Thavarasook C.: *Proceedings of the Mungbean Meeting 90, Chiang Mai, Thailand,* Bangkok, Tropical Agricultural Research Centre, 1991.

Thomas E.: *Fruit Production in St. Kitts and Nevis*, Port of Spain, IICA, 1996.

Vargas E. M., Macaya G., Baudoin J. P. and Rocha O. J.: *Variation in the Content of Phaseolin in Wild Populations of Lima Beans (Phaseolus lunatus L.) in the Central Valley of Costa Rica*. Plant Genetic Resources Newsletter, 2000.

Webb M.: *Weed Problems and their Control in Rice, Papaya, Citrus and Sugar cane: a Report to the Belize Plant Protection Service*, United Kingdom, Natural Resources Institute, 1993.

Whealy K.: *The Garden Seed Inventory*, Decorah, Seed Saver Publications, 1988.

Whitwell A.: *Dominica Orchard Crop Management and Research Project: Pest and Disease Management,* United Kingdom, Natural Resources Institute, 1991.

Woolfe Jennifer A.: *The Potato in the Human Diet*, Cambridge, Cambridge University Press, 1989.

Yoshida T.: *Cultivation of Citrus Genetic Resources for Evaluation of Characteristics*, Tokyo, JICA, 1996.

Index

A

Agriculture, 24, 37, 147, 181, 200, 234, 242, 248, 249.
Alternative Medicine, 51, 59, 65, 66, 67, 68, 69, 70, 71, 72, 73, 76, 77, 147, 240.
Apple, 15, 57, 58, 61.
Aromatherapy, 59, 139.
Asparagus, 249.
Ayurvedic, 7, 50, 64, 69, 75, 77, 79, 80, 81, 125, 205, 234, 246, 247, 253.
Ayurvedic Philosophy, 80, 81.

B

Biological Diversity, 27, 29, 31, 211, 228, 241.
Biosphere, 26, 30.
Biotechnology, 105, 239, 244.
Black Pepper, 90.
Botanical Gardens, 28, 203, 213.
Bulbs, 144, 166, 174, 178, 182, 183, 184, 185, 187, 188.

C

Carbohydrates, 95.
Cardamom, 4, 91.
Carrier Oils, 59.
Celery, 15, 16, 19.
Climate, 34, 35, 155, 168.
Climatic Conditions, 39, 225, 226.
Clove, 118, 119.
Coffee, 13, 53, 56, 210.
Commercial Trade, 216, 218.
Commodities, 212.
Consumption, 1, 159, 160, 165, 168, 176, 201, 225.
Cooperation, 33, 148, 154, 218, 219.
Cosmetic, 144, 145, 146, 220.
Crop Maintenance, 131.
Crops, 19, 36, 44, 105, 131, 132, 133, 135, 139, 143, 181, 191, 211, 227, 234, 247, 248.
Culture, 2, 8, 20, 28, 42, 43, 44, 103, 106, 145, 156, 161, 223.

D

Department, 34, 37, 147, 181, 232, 242, 250.
Documentation, 25, 30, 31, 112, 130, 136, 137, 138, 154, 176, 197, 237, 253.
Drug Development, 38, 39, 40, 113, 124, 125.
Drug Discovery, 7, 8, 41, 109, 111, 124, 125.
Drug Research, 30, 72, 108, 113, 127.

E

Ecophysiology, 94, 95.
Ecosystem, 4, 20, 27, 28, 207.
Erosion, 173, 219, 221, 223.
Essential Oil, 135, 136.
Eucalyptus, 54, 211.
Evaluation, 68, 204, 209.
Export, 12, 150, 216, 229, 241.

Extraction, 32, 56, 57, 59, 100, 141, 222, 249.

F

Farmers, 5, 129, 173, 197, 213, 227, 228, 229, 230, 235, 237, 246, 247, 248, 250, 251.
Farming, 183, 197, 227, 228, 233, 235, 236, 237, 248.
Fenugreek, 17, 91.
Fertility, 14, 41, 141.
Fertilizers, 131, 138.
Flowers, 18, 19, 53, 99, 143, 229, 237.
Folk Medicine, 21, 41, 49, 208.
Forestry, 173, 189, 211, 227, 242.
Foundation, 22, 33, 55, 147, 180, 218.
Fruit, 32, 90, 140, 141, 166, 223.

G

Genetic Diversity, 24, 26, 29, 202, 207, 212, 213, 224, 227, 249.
Genetic Engineering, 42.
Genetic Resources, 24, 28, 36.
Germplasm, 211, 213.
Ginger, 25, 88, 90, 91.
Ginkgo, 14, 100, 101, 117, 118, 139.
Ginseng, 13, 43, 97, 98, 106, 139, 142, 147, 151, 152.
Grapefruit, 60, 73.
Grasses, 4, 21.
Grassland, 173, 174, 181, 182, 183, 199.
Guidelines, 33, 129, 130, 136, 138, 197, 214, 226, 247, 252.

H

Harvest, 34, 38, 44, 103, 107, 130, 132, 133, 137, 138, 148, 149, 150, 151, 152, 154, 155, 171, 175, 179, 186, 187, 188, 191, 192, 206, 217, 224, 225, 247, 252.
Herbal Drugs, 8, 21, 106, 113, 120, 123, 125, 222, 252.
Herbal Tinctures, 56, 57.
Herbalism, 49, 50, 61.
Herbicides, 131, 132, 138.
Homoeopathy, 4, 81, 83, 86, 87, 88.
Hormones, 11, 73, 95.
Horticulture, 37, 94, 203.
Humidity, 132, 136.

I

Import, 205, 239.
Indigenous Medicinal Plants, 164, 173, 183, 192, 194, 197, 200.
Indigenous Medicines, 156, 161, 169, 190, 192, 194, 198.
Infrastructure, 30, 37, 193, 195, 230.
Insects, 50, 51, 133.
Institute, 28, 30, 33, 37, 61, 73, 83, 107, 173, 180, 233, 240.
Institutional Support, 194, 232.
Institutions, 5, 30, 36, 71, 199, 215, 217, 219, 234, 235, 237, 240.
Intellectual Property Rights, 218, 229.
International Trade, 140, 150, 152, 154, 202, 203, 204, 205, 206, 212, 216, 217, 238.
Involvement, 27, 114, 202, 209, 214, 251.

Irrigation, 102, 131.
Islands, 102, 210.

L

Laboratory, 8, 30, 80, 97, 98, 107, 126, 229, 238.
Leaf, 15, 54, 55, 90, 100, 103, 117, 134.
Lemon, 12, 15, 32, 61.
Library, 69, 114, 234.
Literature, 3, 8, 64, 80, 97, 126, 195.

M

Maintenance, 26, 27, 105, 131, 211, 249.
Market Materials, 180.
Market Segments, 156, 163, 198.
Marketing, 35, 93, 153, 187, 193, 194, 197, 202, 208, 218, 230, 231, 233, 234, 235, 239.
Medicinal Plant Markets, 195, 196, 199.

Methodology, 34, 47, 82, 245.
Microarrays, 108, 109, 110, 111, 112, 113, 114, 115, 117, 120, 122, 123, 124, 125, 126, 127.
Moisture, 132, 185.
Monitoring, 117, 123, 252.

N

National Consumption, 159, 160.
National Parks, 26, 27, 30, 32.
Natural Habitats, 236, 248, 249, 251.
Natural Medicines Market, 240.
Network, 26, 27, 28, 36, 150, 213, 235, 243, 245.
Nutrients, 95, 99.

O

Oils, 4, 52, 54, 58, 59, 134, 135.
Operation, 30, 43, 150, 158, 215, 248.
Organic Farming, 248.
Organic Status, 246.
Organisations, 31, 34, 35, 37, 213, 218, 219, 252.

P

Parameters, 38, 46, 47, 107, 214.
Parks, 26, 27, 28, 29, 30, 32, 179.
Parsley, 16, 18.
Pathology, 52, 84.
Pepper, 25, 88, 89, 90, 91.
Performance, 74, 97, 100, 236.
Pest Control, 133, 134, 136.
Pharmacogenomics, 113, 120, 124.
Plant Protection, 131, 132, 138.
Plant Tissue, 28.
Plantations, 12, 173, 181.
Pollination, 51.
Polymorphism, 105, 122, 124.
Pomegranate, 17.
Popularity, 51, 84, 162, 182.
Post Harvest, 38, 107.
Potential Production, 177, 178, 180.
Powdered Herbs, 58.
Preservation, 26, 28, 237.
Prevention, 19, 79, 85, 129.
Priorities, 25, 45, 194, 198.
Projections, 163.
Promotion, 153, 211, 233, 234, 247.
Propagation Techniques, 42.
Protein, 109, 110, 115, 118, 123.
Proteins, 55, 95, 109, 110, 120, 121.
Pukka Herbs, 246, 247, 248, 249, 250, 251.

R

Rainfall, 24, 133.
Resource Management, 174, 192, 201, 202, 249.
Rice, 59, 91.
Rose, 12, 18, 19, 68.
Rosemary, 19, 20, 139.
Roses, 17, 18, 19, 20.
Rotation, 131.
Rural Development, 234.

S

Sanctuaries, 26, 27, 29, 30, 32.
Security, 21, 149, 250.
Shrubs, 21, 28, 139, 144.
Situ Conservation, 26, 27, 28, 30, 34, 203, 213, 214, 232.
Society, 2, 3, 24, 165, 192, 194, 195, 201.
Soil, 98, 99, 104, 131, 132, 133, 141, 235, 246, 247, 249, 250.
Soil Association, 246, 247, 250.
Soils, 131, 132.
Stem, 22, 43, 102.
Storage, 37, 38, 97, 130, 132, 134, 135, 136, 141, 157, 159, 193, 234, 237.
Strategies, 25, 35, 108, 192, 203, 208, 237.
Structure, 28, 52, 109, 112, 121, 125, 205, 235.
Succulents, 144, 185.
Supplements, 1, 50, 59, 64, 69, 77, 239.
Sustainable Agriculture, 249.
Sustainable Management, 27, 154.
Symptoms, 14, 60, 72, 76, 80, 84, 86, 87, 88, 103, 236.

T

Teas, 52, 53, 54, 56, 58, 77, 153.
Temperature, 95, 134, 135, 141.
Tissue Culture, 28, 44, 103, 106.
Tissues, 42, 81, 95, 118.
Toxicology, 84, 120, 124.
Transport, 133, 135, 136, 169, 176, 179, 186, 188, 193, 243.
Tubers, 13, 90, 183, 184, 187.

U

Unani, 5, 23, 24, 46, 68, 71, 84, 85, 86, 88, 222, 231, 236.
University, 49, 52, 67, 141, 147.

V

Variations, 44, 126.
Vegetables, 228.
Vegetation, 4, 21, 146, 182, 187, 210, 211, 249, 252.
Vision, 200.
Vitamins, 51, 55, 73.

W

Weeds, 52, 132.
Welfare, 37, 107, 137, 148, 191, 194, 202.
Wildlife, 29, 129.

❑❑❑